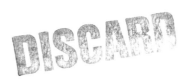

Encyclopedia of
Health

THIRD EDITION

First Aid—Comprehensive Index

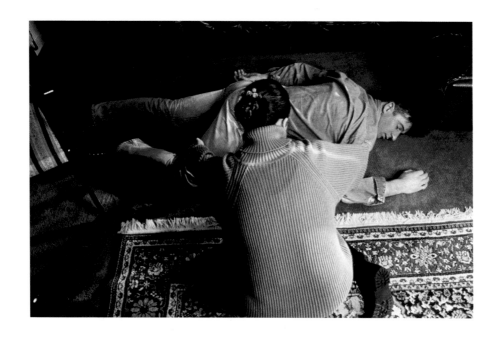

Marshall Cavendish

NEW YORK • TORONTO • LONDON • SYDNEY

Marshall Cavendish
99 White Plains Road
Tarrytown, NY 10591
Website: www.marshallcavendish.com

Brown Partworks Limited
Editor: Anne Hildyard
Associate Editors: Claire Cross, Clare Hill
Editorial Director: Lindsey Lowe
Designers: Matthew Greenfield,
Dax Fullbrook, Seth Grimbly
Picture Research: Susannah Jayes
Index Editor: Kay Ollerenshaw

Library of Congress Cataloging-in-Publication Data

Encyclopedia of health.-- 3rd ed., [rev. & updated].
    p.cm.
    Previously published under the title: The Marshall Cavendish
encyclopedia of health (14 vols.).
    Includes bibliographical references and index.
    ISBN 0-7614-7347-5 (set)
    ISBN 0-7614-7363-7 (vol. 16)

    1. Medicine, Popular--Encyclopedias. 2. Health--Encyclopedias.
1. Marshall Cavendish Corporation. II. Marshall Cavendish encyclopedia
of health.
    RC81.A2 E52 2003
        610'.3--dc21   2001028883

Printed and bound in Italy
07 06 05 04 03 02 7 6 5 4 3 2 1

CONTENTS

First Aid

CONTENTS

First aid is a valuable skill. It provides you with knowledge of how to deal with the most common medical emergencies. The initial treatment may be vital. The aim of first aid is to keep the patient alive, to protect him or her from further injury, and not to make the situation worse by your intervention. The victim should be kept safe until trained medical personnel arrive to take over. Be as reassuring as possible. The priorities when giving first aid are to make sure the patient is breathing and to perform rescue breathing if necessary. Next, try to stop bleeding and treat the patient if he or she is unconscious. Immobilize fractures, treat burns, dress wounds, and minimize the effects of shock. Ensure that you have your family physician's phone number handy, and that you know how to call emergency services in your area.

The following section gives basic information about first aid. However, many of the techniques of first aid can best be learned by taking a first aid course taught by qualified personnel. Check with your local hospital or Red Cross chapter for details about courses.

Bites and Stings

- All bites and stings need different treatment
- Animal bites need to be washed thoroughly
- Some people are allergic to bites and stings
- Bee stingers have to be removed
- If in doubt, call the emergency number

Make sure you...

DO clean any bite or sting with clean, warm water and, if possible, soap that does not contain perfume or detergent. Then gently dab the wound with a mild antiseptic.

DO reassure the victim of a snakebite. Remind them that many people have been bitten by poisonous snakes and lived. Get the victim to describe the snake—it will help a doctor to prescribe the right treatment quickly.

DO apply calamine lotion or cream to insect bites or stings, including those from gnats and fleas.

DO get medical help quickly in the following instances:

1 Stings inside the mouth

2 Patients known to be allergic

3 Signs of shock—pallor, sweating, collapse, and breathing difficulties

4 Stinging by swarms of insects

5 If there is severe bleeding and you cannot stop the bleeding yourself

DO take care when you remove a bee stinger. Make sure you do not break or squeeze the venom sac and release more venom into the wound.

DON'T treat a snakebite by cutting the area, trying to suck out the venom, or by applying ice or a tourniquet. These treatments are all dangerous. Instead, call the emergency number so they can prepare the correct antivenin.

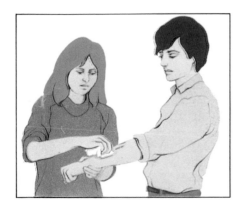

1 *Treat animal bites like ordinary wounds (see page 916). If bleeding is minor, wash wound and cover it. Consult a doctor.*

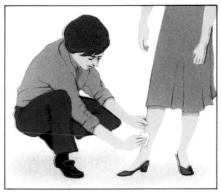

2 *To treat a snakebite, wash the wound. To stop the venom from spreading, keep the victim still with the wound below heart level. Call the emergency number.*

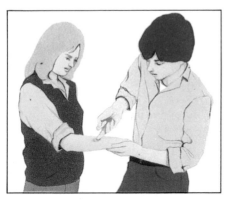

3 *Bee stingers left in the wound continue to pump in venom after the insect has gone. Scrape the stinger out sideways with a fingernail or plastic card.*

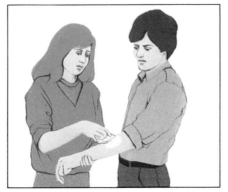

4 *Clean marine life stings and rinse well in salt water. Apply a cold pack and then call the emergency number. Try to find out what caused the stings.*

Prickly plants

- Plants with prickles and thorns can break the surface of the skin, which can lead to a tetanus infection. Pull out thorns with fine tweezers. If they are embedded, apply a dressing and see a doctor.

- Wash stings from poisonous plants with hot water and soap. Calamine lotion or cream relieves the itching.

- Some cactus plants leave hundreds of fine needles embedded in the skin. They can be very difficult to pull out and they are extremely uncomfortable if left in the skin. To remove the needles, press an adhesive bandage or a piece of tape onto the affected area. Pull off the adhesive bandage and the sticky surface should remove the prickles with it.

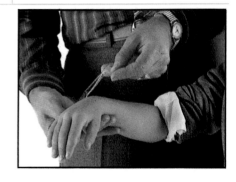

Take note

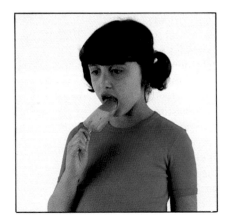

• If a victim is stung inside the mouth, get medical aid immediately. If the mouth swells, breathing can be seriously impaired. While you wait for help, minimize the swelling with cold mouthwashes, ice cubes, or popsicles.

• The risk of infection is high with any animal bite, so always consult a doctor. If there is a risk that the attacking animal was rabid, go to a hospital immediately or call the emergency number. Report the animal to animal control personnel.

• Poisonous spiders and scorpions live in dark, out-of-the-way places. Their bites may cause painful swellings, nausea and vomiting, and difficulty breathing and swallowing. Wash the victim's wound and apply a cold pack. Get medical care to administer antivenin.

• Remove a bee stinger by scraping it off with something firm, such as a credit card or fingernail. Do not use tweezers to remove the stinger—pinching it may release more venom.

• Ticks are parasites that feed on humans and other warm-blooded vertebrates. Some ticks are harmless, but because others transmit disease, a tick must be removed promptly. Suffocate it with mineral oil or petroleum jelly, then grasp near the head with tweezers and pull the tick out carefully, ensuring that the head is completely removed. Apply an antiseptic to the wound. Consult a doctor immediately if fever, rash, aches, or pains occur days or weeks after the bite.

What next?

1 Make sure that the patient does not scratch the affected area of the bite or sting. The irritation and itching can be very annoying, but scratching or rubbing help spread the venom and increase the chances of infection. A cold compress, calamine lotion, or antiseptic ointment can help to reduce any irritation.

2 Any pain resulting from bites and stings usually disappears naturally within an hour or two. Aspirin or acetaminophen may speed up pain relief. Do not give aspirin to children.

3 The risk of infection is high, particularly with bites. If there is increased pain, swelling, redness, discharge, swollen lymph nodes, or fever over the next few days, consult the doctor. Always visit a doctor in the case of animal bites.

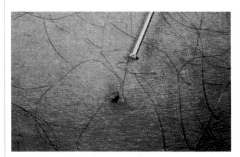

4 Shock can be caused by any bite or sting, no matter how minor, especially if the victim is elderly or very young. Any patient may suffer an allergic reaction to the venom, or just be very frightened. Always treat for shock (see page 910). Get help as quickly as possible, but, if at all possible, do not leave the patient alone. Keep the affected area absolutely still.

5 Although all plant and animal poisons are different, they each provoke the release of histamine, a substance that can produce symptoms varying from rashes to serious breathing difficulties. Doctors may decide to administer an antihistamine to counteract the effects of the poison. Also check whether the victim is up to date with immunizations for tetanus and inform the doctor of this.

A deer tick (left) can be as small as the head of a pin. It is possible to get Lyme disease from a tick bite, so it is essential to remove it. Use tweezers or, if you use your fingers, wash your hands at once.

Use a credit card (below) to scrape off bee stingers. Wash, cover, and apply a cold pack.

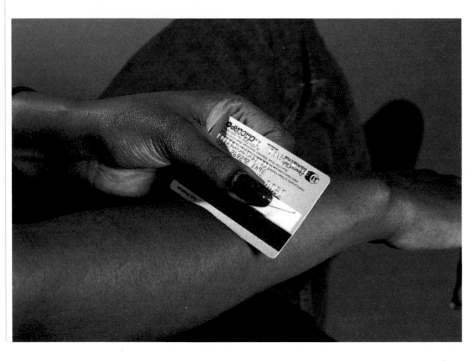

Bleeding

- Apply pressure to the wound with a pad to stop the bleeding
- Unless there is a fracture, raise the injured part to diminish the force of the blood flow at the injury
- Maintain pressure even after a clot has formed
- Move the limb as little as possible—there may be further injuries

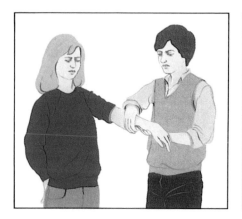

1 *Stop the bleeding by applying firm pressure to the wound. If possible, avoid direct contact with the patient's blood by using any available material (such as a handkerchief) as a pad.*

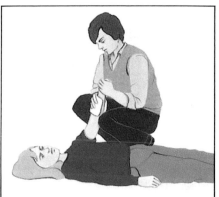

2 *Lie the patient down and raise the bleeding part above the level of the patient's heart, if you are certain there is not a broken bone, and if this does not cause any pain. Continue to apply pressure.*

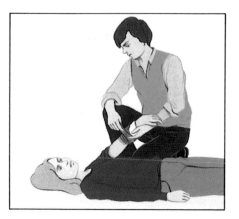

3 *Maintain pressure and find a belt, scarf, or tie to act as a bandage. Wrap it tight enough to maintain pressure but not so tight that it cuts off circulation, and secure with a firm knot over the wound.*

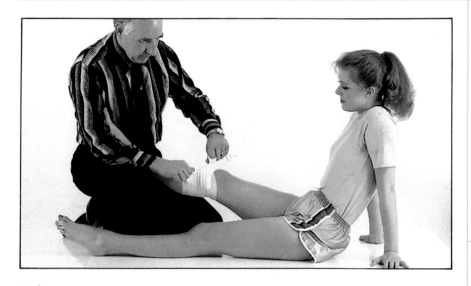

Make sure you...

DO tie the bandage very firmly, but never apply a tourniquet.

DO get your patient to lie or sit down. Ensure they are not disturbed.

DO make sure that the patient is calm and reassured before you get help.

DON'T waste time washing your hands or finding dressings. Speed is more important—the risk of hemorrhage is greater than the risk of infection.

DON'T ask the patient to help you by using his or her hand to exert pressure—he or she may be too weak.

Take note

- Keep checking for signs of shock. Patients may be faint, pale, cold, sweating, or thirsty. They may have a rapid pulse and shallow breathing rate.

- If any of these signs appear in a patient with no visible injury, there may be internal bleeding. Send for help.

- If a patient vomits blood, it is likely that there is bleeding in the stomach. Get help as soon as possible.

What next?

1 The risk of shock is high when the patient has lost a lot of blood, so keep him or her lightly covered; warming is dangerous; stay with the patient.

2 In cases of severe bleeding, call an ambulance immediately.

3 A patient should lie quietly and avoid any movement until help arrives.

What to do in an emergency

Coughing up blood
Place the patient in the recovery position (see below). If breathing is difficult, prop up on pillows. Get help quickly. If even a small amount of blood is coughed up, it must be reported to a doctor.

Vomiting blood
Place the patient in the recovery position (below). Clean the mouth. Get help urgently. Keep the vomit for the doctor to examine. If red blood is vomited, the bleeding is probably severe and fast.

Internal bleeding
Pain or discomfort can be deceptively slight and because signs and symptoms can take days or weeks to appear, internal bleeding may go unnoticed. It is a life-threatening condition, and if it is suspected, the victim needs to get to the hospital quickly. If the patient shows signs of shock (faintness, pallor, coldness, sweating, thirst, fast and weak pulse and breathing), loosen any tight clothing, then cover the patient. If there is no head, neck, back or leg injury and the victim feels comfortable, place him or her in the shock position(see page 910): lie the victim flat and elevate the feet 20–30 cm (8–12 in.). Do not give anything to eat or drink. Get help immediately.

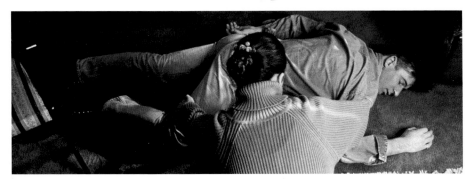

Different types of bleeding

Bleeding from the palm
Raise the patient's arm. Make a thick pad for the patient to clench. Wrap a bandage around the pad and knot it securely at the back of the hand.

Nosebleed
Have the victim sit with the head slightly forward while pinching the nostrils together. If bleeding continues, apply a cold pack to the bridge of the nose.

Bleeding from the tongue
Grip the tongue firmly between finger and thumb with a clean handkerchief. Keep up the pressure for 10 minutes. If the bleeding is severe, make sure blood can drain from the mouth so that the victim can breathe. If the injury is minor, give the person an ice cube to suck.

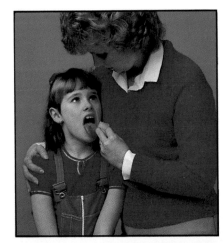

Burns

- If there are flames, smother with a cloth; get medical help
- In the event of less severe burns, immerse affected area in cold water for at least 10 minutes
- Cover burned area with clean, dry dressing and guard against shock
- Lie patient down and phone for ambulance or doctor

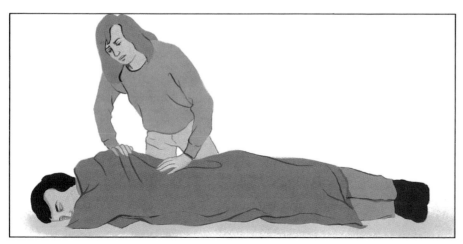

If the victim's clothes are on fire, try to smother the flames by pressing down with a suitably thick cloth, such as a towel, curtain, rug, or jacket. Don't roll the patient around on the floor. Once the fire is out, pull away charred or smoldering cloth if it comes away easily. Otherwise, leave anything sticking to the skin alone to avoid further injury and to ensure that you do not disturb any burns or blisters. Remove rings or any other item that is constricting, as the area may swell up.

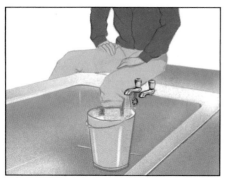

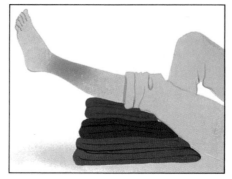

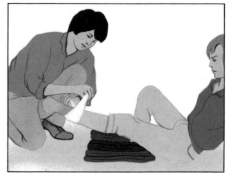

1 *Put the burned limb into cold water to cool it down. Keep the cold water running over the burn. Immerse for at least 10 minutes. Alternatively, cover the area with a thick wet cloth. Keep it damp.*

2 *If the face is burned, have patient sit up. In other severe cases, keep the patient lying down. Elevate a burned limb to reduce swelling. A leg, for instance, can be propped up on pillows.*

3 *Cover the area with a clean, dry protective gauze pad and then bandage or strap it on lightly. Make sure the area is well cooled before you cover it. Do not apply lotions or ointments.*

Take note

- Burns may be caused by moist heat such as steam or boiling liquids. Saturated clothes will continue to burn the skin unless they are taken off quickly. Cool a scalded throat with mouthfuls of cold water or by sucking ice cubes.

- Dry heat burns come from flames or from touching hot objects. Friction can cause burns, and electricity can cause deep burns.

- Corrosive chemicals like strong acids can burn severely. Wash vigorously with cold water and flush for 15 minutes. Get medical help but don't leave the victim.

- A victim who is not in shock can take small amounts of sweetened water to help replace lost body fluids.

- Protect skin with high factor sunscreen. See a doctor if you have bad sunburn.

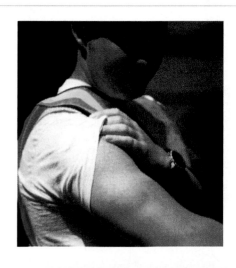

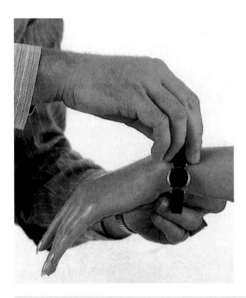

Make sure you...

DO remove anything that might cause constriction if the injury swells.

DO keep a burned limb elevated to reduce swelling.

DON'T roll the victim on the floor to extinguish the flames of burning clothes, just cover the area firmly.

DON'T try to pull away anything that is stuck to the burned area.

DON'T apply cream or ointment to the burned area.

What next?

1 When assessing the injury, note that the surface area of the burn is more significant than the depth.

2 Generally, do not give patients anything by mouth. In the case of burns, you may give the patient about half a glassful of tepid water every 15 or 20 minutes until help arrives. The water may be sweetened slightly, but remember that fluids can cause vomiting if the patient is suffering from shock, which is a serious risk with burn injuries. The liquid helps to replace lost body fluids. If vomiting occurs or if the patient feels nauseous, stop giving fluids.

3 Anyone who has been badly burned should be taken to the hospital as soon as possible. Call an ambulance; it is quicker and allows the patient to remain lying down.

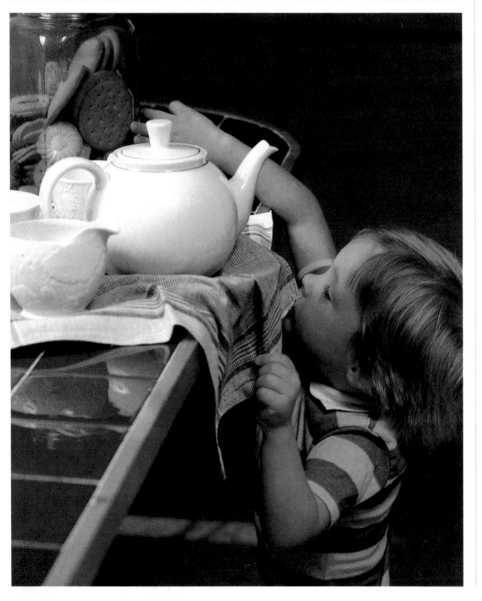

This child is about to suffer a serious but common household injury— a bad burn. Make sure that teapots, saucepans, and other containers of hot liquid are kept out of the reach of inquisitive hands, away from the edge of a table or work surface. Do not place hot containers on mats, tablecloths, or dish towels where they can be pulled off easily. Never leave cookies or candy near hot drinks. A child will not understand the danger and, trying to reach the cookies, may pull the boiling liquid over himself or herself.

Choking

- As long as the patient can talk and cough vigorously, do not interfere
- If the patient cannot cough, try back blows
- If the object does not dislodge, use abdominal thrusts (the Heimlich maneuver)
- If the patient collapses, begin rescue breathing
- When airways are completely blocked, try to remove the obstruction

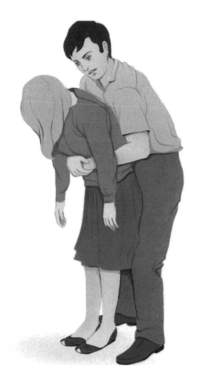

1 *If the patient cannot talk or cough, start performing abdominal thrusts (the Heimlich maneuver). Continue using abdominal thrusts until the obstruction is dislodged or the patient passes out.*

To perform the Heimlich maneuver, stand behind the person who is choking and wrap your arms around his or her waist. With one hand, make a fist. Place the thumb side of the fist against the victim's abdomen, just above the navel. Put your other hand over your fist and then pull your hands inward, giving quick, upward thrusts into the victim's abdomen. Continue giving the thrusts until the object blocking the airway is dislodged and the victim begins to breathe. If the person stops breathing, start rescue breathing immediately (see page 908) and send for help.

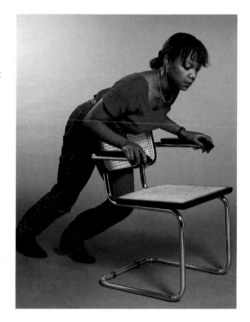

If you are alone and choking, give yourself abdominal thrusts by pressing your abdomen onto a firm object, like a chair.

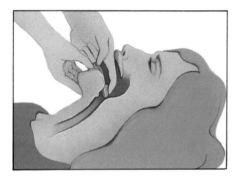

2 *If the patient's airway is completely obstructed and you cannot get air into the patient's lungs by rescue breathing, you must try to find and remove the object. Place a curved finger into the mouth and probe the area gently. Be careful not to push the finger straight in as you might move the object deeper into the throat. Start at the side of the cheek, moving the finger to the back of the mouth; then hook the finger forward to dislodge the object. Pull it out of the mouth quickly, in case the patient sucks it back into the throat again.*

Take note

If a baby or toddler is choking, put the child, facing downward, across your forearm. Put your other arm on top of the infant, making sure that the infant's head is lower than his or her chest. With the heel of your hand, give five back blows between the infant's shoulder blades. If this does not work, turn the child face up and give four chest thrusts as if for external cardiac compression. (See CPR, page 915). Continue giving back blows and chest thrusts until the infant can breathe or cough. Make sure the child is examined by a doctor urgently.

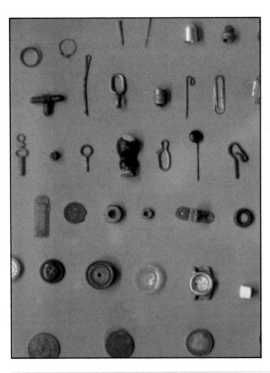

Make sure you...

Stay with the patient, even if he is able to speak and cough.

Keep the patient calm. Anxiety can increase the tension of the muscles, causing the obstruction to be held more tightly.

Make very certain that toys are safe. Avoid those with small parts that can be easily removed.

Keep all small objects out of the reach of babies and toddlers. Small children are particularly likely to put objects into their mouth.

Let the patient try to dislodge the object by coughing before trying backslaps and abdominal thrusts.

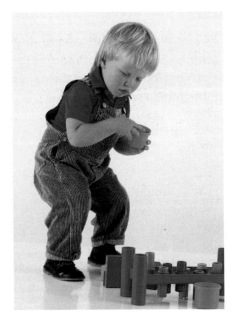

Make sure children only play with toys that they cannot swallow (above).

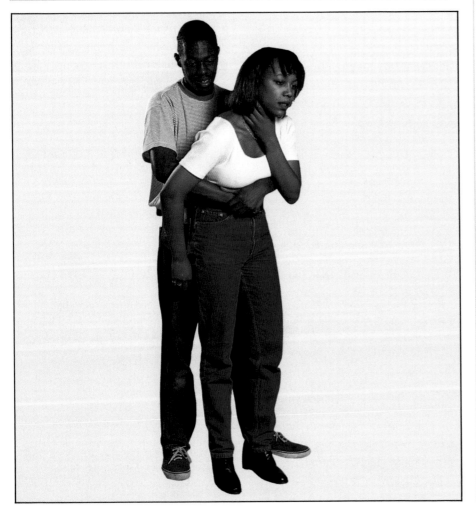

What next?

1 When something is swallowed the wrong way, it can obstruct the back of the throat or move a little further down and block the windpipe.

2 If the obstructing object becomes free and moves into the patient's mouth, seize it and pull it out quickly. Otherwise, the patient's next sudden breath might suck it back again.

3 If the patient feels faint or vomits, put him or her in the recovery position (see page 895).

4 The person who has choked should be examined by a doctor if blows or abdominal thrusts have been used.

Above left: An array of objects that might be swallowed and then become stuck in the windpipe.

Left: Use abdominal thrusts to dislodge the object only after you have tried to remove it by using hard blows between the shoulder blades.

Convulsions

- When patient collapses and lies rigid before a convulsion, push head back, loosen clothes
- Don't try to control thrashing limbs, surround patient with pillows
- When jerking stops, keep the patient's head back
- If uninjured and safe to move, place the patient in the recovery position

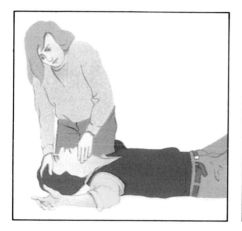

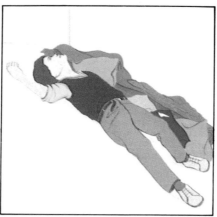

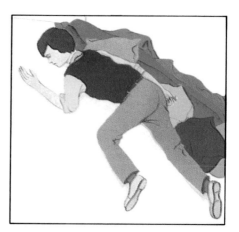

1 *Before the convulsion, clear the airway by pushing the head back gently. Loosen any tight clothing, particularly around the neck. Remember that the patient may have injured himself or herself when he or she fell.*

2 *When convulsions start, do not attempt to control the thrashing limbs. Instead, surround the patient with soft buffers to protect him or her from self-inflicted injuries and move dangerous objects out of the way.*

3 *The patient stops jerking and relaxes, but remains unconscious. Keep the head tilted back; look for injuries. If it is safe to move the victim, put him or her on their side in the recovery position. Stay with the patient until he or she recovers.*

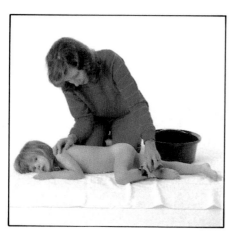

Fever convulsions

A small child developing a high fever may react with a brief convulsion.

- Stay by the child's side; tip the head back; put the child in the recovery position. Remove child's clothes and cool down with a cold, wet sponge.

- When the attack ends, keep the child lightly covered.

- If there are any complications, dial 911.

Take note

- An epileptic attack or a child's feverish convulsion is alarming, but usually such seizures are short-lived.

- Attacks vary from patient to patient. Most often, they come without any warning. The patient becomes unconscious; he or she may cry out and not be aware he or she has done so.

- The patient begins jerking or thrashing the limbs and face. This part of the attack can last 30 seconds. The patient may froth at the mouth; hold his or her breath; bite his or her tongue; or may be incontinent.

- When the patient stops jerking, he or she will remain unconscious for several minutes. When conscious again, the victim may be drowsy at first and may dislike fuss around him or her and want to take care of himself or herself.

Make sure you...

DO loosen any tight clothing when the convulsion starts. Push the patient's head back to make sure that he or she does not choke during the seizure.

DON'T force open the mouth or put anything in it, including your fingers.

DON'T try to control jerking or thrashing limbs, but do try to protect the victim from self-inflicted injuries.

DON'T send for an ambulance unless the patient has not regained consciousness after 15 minutes.

Electric Shock

- **Turn the electricity off at the outlet**
- **Do not touch the victim**
- **Check that the victim is breathing**
- **Send for help urgently**

General points

- The vast majority of electrical injuries occur in the home.

- Do not touch a victim until he or she has been separated from the current, or the electricity supply has been turned off. If you do touch the victim, you may receive a shock as well.

- It is vital that you do not put yourself in danger. Do not touch anything that is in contact with a wire. Try to move the victim away from a live wire, using a wooden brush handle or chair. If you cannot safely turn the power off, call the power company or 911 immediately.

- Once the victim is free, keep the head tilted back and the airway open. Monitor the victim's breathing and heartbeat. If necessary, start to give the victim rescue breathing, CPR, or bleeding control (see pages 894, 908, 915) immediately. Check for serious injuries, deal with those, then give first aid for entry and exit burns.

- Call for help immediately. Stay with the victim. Watch for signs of collapse (whiteness and sweating) until the ambulance arrives. Place victim in the recovery position (see page 895). Stay with the victim until help arrives.

What next?

1 After calling an ambulance, keep a close eye on the patient. Do not allow people to crowd around him or her. Make sure he or she is comfortable, and keep a watch for signs of deterioration.

2 If the victim stops breathing at any time, he or she needs rescue breathing either until he or she starts breathing again, or until the ambulance arrives.

3 If the victim's breathing and heartbeat recover, place him or her in the recovery position (see page 895).

Make sure you...

DON'T handle any switches, plugs, or electrical appliances with wet hands.

DON'T touch the skin of someone who is being electrocuted.

DON'T move a victim of electric shock unless it is dangerous not to do so.

DO check the victim's airway, breathing, and circulation. If necessary, give first aid for unconsciousness (page 914).

DO check the victim for any injuries and give first aid for entry and exit burns.

DO try to prevent shock and cover the victim with a blanket or coat.

DO stay with the person until the emergency services arrive.

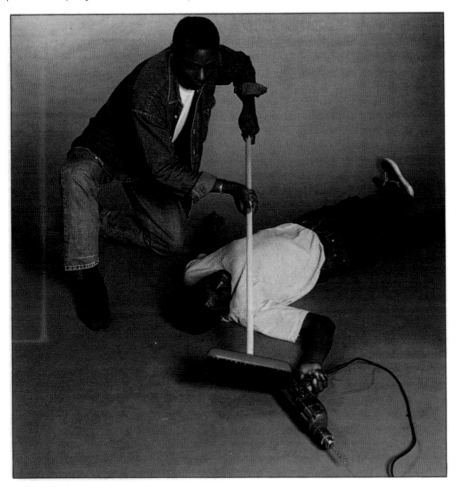

If you discover the victim of an electric shock, do not touch him or her until he or she is separated from the current. You could receive an equally forceful shock. Turn off the electricity supply at once. If this is not possible, stand on a dry, non-conducting material such as a rubber mat or paper before pushing the live apparatus away. Do not use any object that is metal or wet. The wooden handle of a broom is ideal. Once the victim is free, check whether or not he or she is breathing—the patient may need urgent rescue breathing.

Exposure and Cold

- Exposure to cold can cause lasting damage to the body's tissues
- Complications associated with exposure include frostbite and hypothermia
- The extremities—nose, earlobes, fingers, and toes—are most affected
- Any attempt at rapid warming can cause further tissue damage

Exposure

Symptoms of exposure include physical and mental deterioration, decrease in reasoning power, change in mood, slurred speech, shivering and cramping, followed by possible collapse. Once these symptoms are detected, stop the patient from moving, but get them to shelter. Remove any wet clothing and replace with blankets, a sleeping bag, or fresh clothing. Cover the patient's head and face, but leave the mouth, nose, and eyes free. If the patient is conscious give warm, sweet drinks. Do not give alcohol under any circumstances; it widens the blood vessels of the skin and promotes heat loss from the body.

Frostbite

Tissues under the skin may freeze in intense cold. The formation of minute ice particles disrupts the blood supply. Clumps of red blood cells form that then block the vessels. Where tissue is numb and white and frostbite is suspected, remove wet clothing and constricting objects (such as rings) from the affected part. Apply a dry, protective cover after gently dabbing away any moisture. If practical, rewarm hands or feet by immersing for at least 30 minutes in warm, not hot, water (100–105°F). Rewarm other areas by applying warm (not hot) compresses. Otherwise, use a warm blanket. Do not rub the area.

Hypothermia

An adult patient with hypothermia is extremely cold all over with puffy skin that is white or blue. A child, however, will look pink. The heartbeat in both adults and children will be slow and weak. If these symptoms are present, keep the patient in bed in the recovery position. Cover the patient with blankets, but keep them loose. Do not use hot water bottles or an electric blanket, as excessive heat may do more damage. Make sure that all open windows are shut and then warm the room with any available heater. If the patient is alert and conscious and can swallow easily, give warm, nonalcoholic drinks.

Make sure you...

DO cover your head in extreme cold to protect against loss of body heat.

DO provide warm sleeping conditions for both the young and the elderly. They are vulnerable to low temperatures.

DO wear suitable protective clothing outside in extremely cold conditions. On long trips, take high energy foods, such as granola and glucose, and containers of hot drinks.

DON'T smoke or drink alcohol.

When traveling or camping somewhere where there is a risk of exposure to cold, damp weather, make sure to take a supply of light thermal blankets as well as a foil thermal blanket for emergencies, as this is an efficient way of retaining body heat after exposure to the cold. Warm up in front of a fire in cases of chill and mild exposure, for example, after a soaking. However, never put victims of severe exposure or frostbite in front of fires, as rapid heating may cause tissue damage.

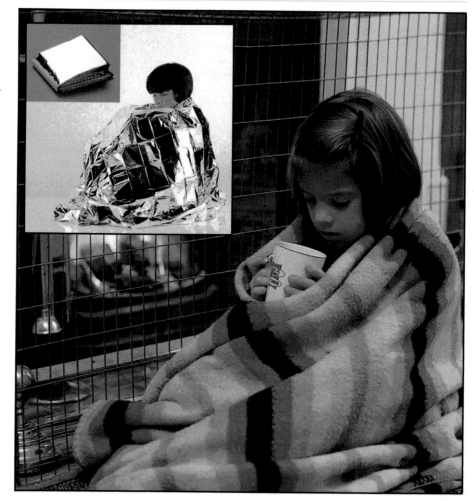

Falls

- Do not try to pick the patient up immediately, but check for injuries
- If a fracture is suspected, do not move the patient
- If no injuries are present, help the patient onto all fours, placing a chair in front for support
- Get the patient to bend one knee and lean forward
- Move to one side, then help the patient to push up

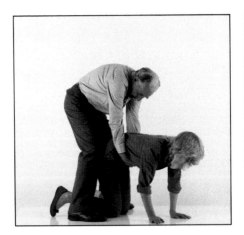 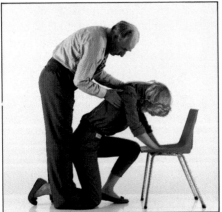 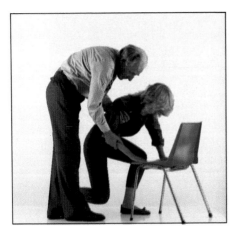

1 *Clear the area of any objects that could get in the way. If the patient can use their arms and legs, turn their face down. Stand over her legs. Hold onto the hip regions and help them onto all fours.*

2 *Place a chair or stool in front of him or her. Help him or her put her hands on the seat. Get him or her to bend one knee and lean forward carefully. You will still be straddling his or her legs.*

3 *Move to one side of the victim. Put one hand in the armpit of that side and the other on the elbow. Now help him or her to push up, using the chair as extra support. Lift as gently as possible.*

Make sure you...

DO examine the patient carefully for injuries; give first aid where appropriate.

DO reassure the patient and stay near.

DON'T attempt to move the patient if there is the slightest chance that there may be a fracture. Let him or her lie without moving until expert help arrives.

DON'T try to pick him or her up at once. Advise him or her to lie still.

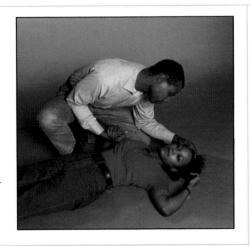

Take note

- Is the patient injured in any way? Establish that he or she is conscious. Ask if there is any pain. Check for bleeding, wounds, and for fractures.

- Is it safe to move the patient? It is not advisable if there is any chance of a fracture. A fall from a height, a blow to the back, or pain in the back or neck might mean a fractured spine. Make the patient comfortable, but do not move him or her. Send for medical help at once.

- Most patients will be able to get up by themselves. The elderly and the weak may need help.

What next?

1 Call a doctor if the patient's condition is uncertain, especially if he or she has grown weaker, if there has been a change in mental attitude, if he or she has a head injury or has lost consciousness.

2 If the patient's legs are weak, get him or her to sit on the floor and place a low stool behind. Help to put his or her hands on the seat and bend forward; the patient can then use his or her arms to push up and sit on the stool. Put a chair behind the stool and repeat the maneuver to get the person to sit on it.

3 Stay with the patient until they begin to feel better. If you have any cause for concern or the patient begins to complain of pain or other symptoms, seek medical advice. Be calm and reassuring until help arrives.

Fractures

- Keep the patient still; cover with a blanket
- Attend to such injuries as an open wound or bleeding before dealing with the fracture
- If necessary, protect the broken bone
- Stay with the patient, and make him or her comfortable until help arrives

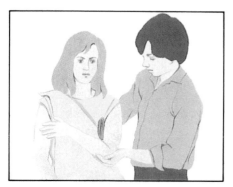

1 *To make an arm sling, support the elbow, keeping the hand raised. Pass the bandage between the chest and arm.*

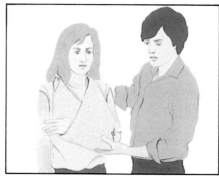

2 *Bring the bandage over the forearm and around the back of neck. Tie the points on the hollow above the collarbone.*

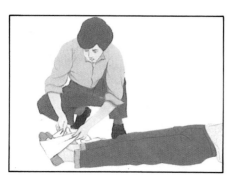

1 *For a figure-eight bandage, place the patient's feet together. Wrap the bandage around the soles of the feet.*

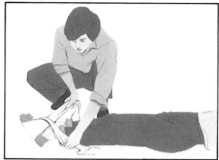

2 *Bring the ends of the bandage to the front. Cross the bandage on the insteps. Carry the ends behind the ankles.*

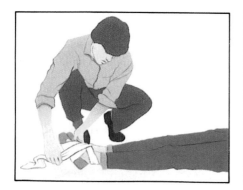

3 *Cross the ends, bring them back to the front of the ankles and cross again. Take ends back under soles. Tie securely.*

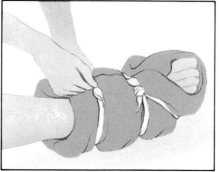

1 *For a foot and ankle bandage, use a flat pillow or folded cloth around the ankle and foot. Secure with bandage strips.*

What next?

- In the case of a broken backbone, the fracture of a vertebra might create loose pieces of bone that could press on the spinal cord, causing permanent paralysis and loss of feeling. Do not move the patient. Let him or her lie as you found him or her and wait for the doctor or ambulance to arrive.

- Meanwhile, make certain the patient cannot move. Try to make him or her comfortable and calm.

- Deciding whether someone has broken a bone can be difficult—many of the classic features are relevant to other injuries, such as sprains. For example, an initial symptom that is quite common is pain; a severe contusion without a break can be extremely painful; and sometimes a major fracture only hurts a little.

- Restricted movement of the injured part and swelling of tissues in the area can be symptomatic of both sprains and fractures. Also, in many fractures the ends of the broken bone are in their correct anatomical position so that the breakage is not always obvious.

Take note

- Unless the patient is in a dangerous situation, warn him or her not to move.

- Look for and control any bleeding. Dress any wounds. Do not try to move the patient if you suspect a neck or spinal injury.

- If expert help is likely to come quickly, let the patient wait, lying quietly, and make him comfortable.

- Protect the patient from shock (see page 910). Place in the shock position only if you are sure that there is no neck, back, or leg injury.

- Protect the patient from the risk of further injury.

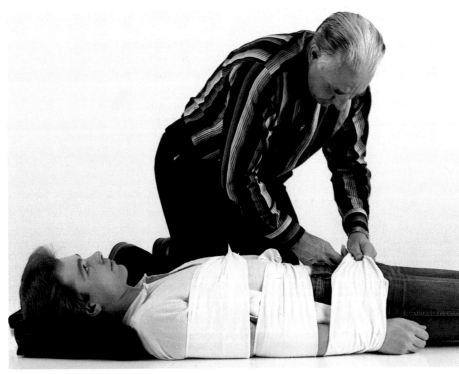

Make sure you...

DO use an uninjured part of the patient's body as a splint (for example, leg to leg, arm to chest) if you have to immobilize a fracture. Whenever possible, move the uninjured part to the injured part.

DO place thick padding, such as absorbent cotton, folded towels, scarves, and socks, to fill spaces between the two parts of the body.

DO tie the parts together carefully and securely. If bandages are not available, improvise with scarves, neckties, or handkerchiefs, for example.

DO tie any knots over the uninjured areas.

DO avoid having a bandage tied directly over a fracture.

To immobilize a fractured arm, put a pad between the arm and body and tie bandages around the upper arm and chest; lower arm and chest; and wrist and thighs (above). If the person can remain upright, support with an arm sling (below).

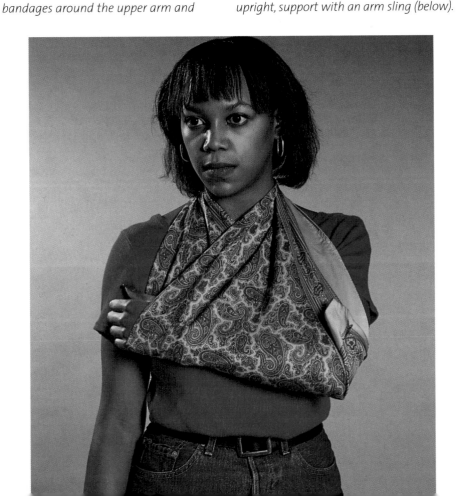

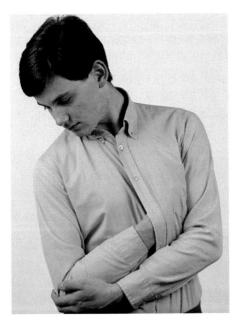

If a triangular bandage is not available, an adequate emergency sling can be rapidly improvised from clothing. The patient's arm can be placed inside his shirt, supported by the fastened buttons. A necktie can be used, or the hem of a jacket can be turned up over the fractured arm and pinned to the lapel.

Heart Attack

- **Call an ambulance immediately**
- **Place the patient in a resting position**
- **Keep the upper part of the body raised**
- **Loosen any tight clothing at neck and waist**
- **If breathing stops, start rescue breathing**
- **Keep patient warm by covering with a blanket**

When a person suffers a heart attack, prompt action is vital. Perform the following in the order shown.

1 *Call, or send someone to call, for an ambulance immediately. Tell the operator what has happened.*

2 *Place the patient upright in a resting position in bed, on a sofa, or in an armchair. This makes it easier to breathe.*

3 *Loosen restrictive clothing at the neck, chest, and waist.*

4 *If the patient appears very breathless, sit him up against a bedrest banked with pillows. An improvised prop can be made from a light chair set upside down.*

5 *If there is nothing suitable to prop the patient against, use your body as a prop for him or her to lean on.*

6 *Keep the sufferer well covered up, but loosely. Open the window so that the room is well ventilated.*

7 *Reassure the patient that medical help is on its way.*

8 *Remain with the patient to comfort him, but prevent others from crowding around.*

9 *If the patient loses consciousness and stops breathing, begin rescue breathing at once (see page 908).*

Take note

- The blood supply to the heart muscle comes from small arteries. If these vessels have become so narrow that they cannot provide the extra blood needed during exertion, the result is a pain in the chest known as angina. The pain is vicelike and sometimes spreads to the neck, shoulders, and arms.

- During a severe heart attack, a clot blocking one of the arteries cuts off the blood from part of the heart muscle. Known as coronary thrombosis, the attack results in intense pain. The patient collapses, is pale, sweats, and has a fast, weak, and often irregular pulse.

- In some cases, symptoms are mild and similar to those of indigestion. When in doubt, treat as a heart attack.

- Acute heart failure is different from the conditions listed above. Here, a weakened heart muscle suddenly stops its normal pumping action. Blood flowing into the heart from the lungs is not propelled forward fully, and the lungs become congested. There is no pain, but the patient may cough up watery, blood-tinged sputum, and saliva may appear around the mouth in bubbles.

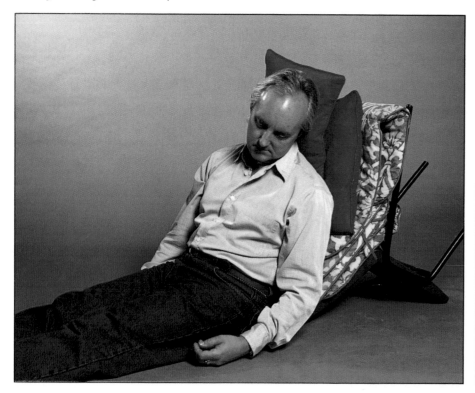

What next?

1 Following treatment and recovery, the patient may be at risk for further heart attacks.

2 Heart patients will increase their chances of living a normal lifespan if they follow the doctor's advice closely.

3 Particular attention should be paid to diet. Smokers should quit. They are at greater risk of heart attacks.

4 The patient should follow the doctor's instructions about starting an exercise program and following a healthy, low-fat diet.

Poisoning

- Call an ambulance and the Poison Control Center
- If unconscious, put in the recovery position
- If the person is not breathing, start rescue breathing

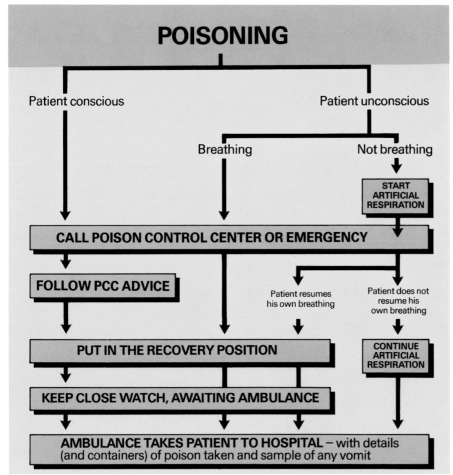

POISONING

Patient conscious — Patient unconscious

Breathing — Not breathing

START ARTIFICIAL RESPIRATION

CALL POISON CONTROL CENTER OR EMERGENCY

FOLLOW PCC ADVICE

Patient resumes his own breathing — Patient does not resume his own breathing

PUT IN THE RECOVERY POSITION

CONTINUE ARTIFICIAL RESPIRATION

KEEP CLOSE WATCH, AWAITING AMBULANCE

AMBULANCE TAKES PATIENT TO HOSPITAL – with details (and containers) of poison taken and sample of any vomit

Follow the above flow diagram to help you decide what action to take in poisoning incidents, where the patient is conscious or unconscious.

Pesticides

- These are very variable in their action. The more dangerous ones can cause harm if swallowed, breathed in, or absorbed through the skin.

- The effects of pesticide poisoning can be cumulative, causing headaches, fatigue, muscle aches, weakness, sweating, vomiting, difficulty in, or even cessation of, breathing.

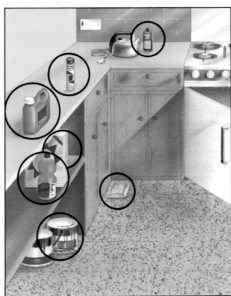

Take note

- It is important to find out quickly which poison the patient has swallowed. Then telephone your local Poison Control Center immediately.

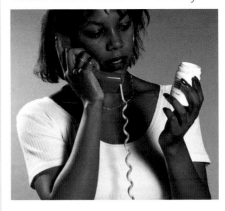

- Check the victim's breathing and pulse. Give rescue breathing if necessary.

- Do not give the victim anything to eat or drink unless the doctor approves.

- Do not try to make the patient vomit unless the doctor instructs you to.

- Give any containers of the suspected substance to the hospital. They will be able to provide appropriate treatment if they know what the substance is.

- Watch the patient in case he vomits, loses consciousness, or stops breathing.

What next?

1 Remember that all poisonous, or potentially poisonous, substances should be kept in locked cupboards out of a child's reach.

2 Ensure that poisons are labeled clearly and in their original containers. The label may give instructions about what to do in an emergency.

The kitchen is a dangerous place for children. Cleaning products, aerosols, detergents, rodent repellants, and paints are poisonous if inhaled, spilled on the skin, or injested accidentally.

Rescue Breathing

- Hold the patient's head back
- Pinch patient's nose and take a deep breath
- Place your mouth over patient's and breathe into patient's mouth
- Check for pulse
- Repeat procedure until breathing resumes

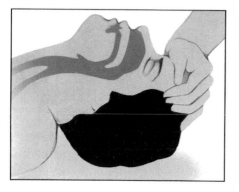

1 *Lift the patient's neck. Push the head gently back. This opens the airway.*

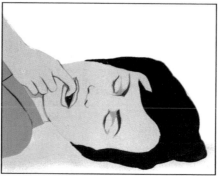

2 *If there is an obstruction, turn the head to one side and clear out the mouth.*

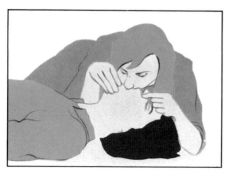

3 *Take a deep breath. Place your mouth over patient's. Blow four quick breaths into the victim's mouth.*

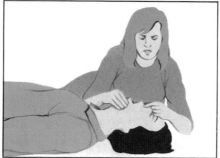

4 *Listen for air leaving the victim's mouth and see if the chest is moving. If there is a pulse, but no breathing, continue.*

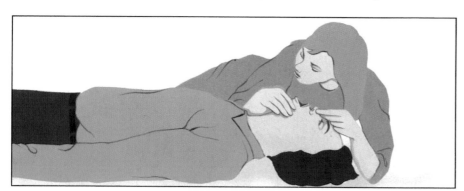

5 *Take another deep breath and blow once into the victim's mouth. Blow hard enough just to raise chest. Give one breath every five seconds (12 per minute)* *and continue until breathing resumes or the emergency services take over. If you suspect a neck, back, or head injury, lift the chin rather than tilting the head back.*

Take note

- If the victim is a young child or baby, open the airway by gently tilting the child's head back. Check breathing before starting rescue breathing. Place your mouth over both the mouth and nose of the child. Do not blow too hard—just enough to raise the chest. Give two slow breaths. If you can feel a pulse, continue giving breaths, one every 3 seconds for a baby, and every 4 seconds for a child.

- If the treatment is interrupted, start again by giving four quick breaths to give an immediate supply of oxygen.

- Check the circulation: place two fingers on the carotid pulse, which is found at the side of the neck just below the jaw.

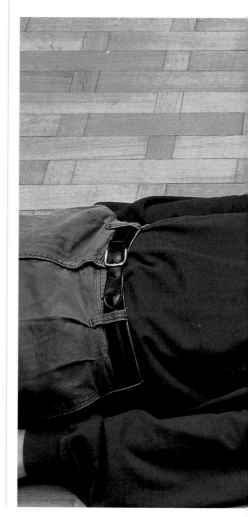

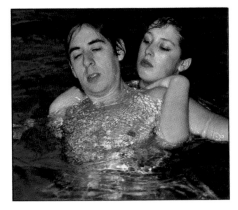 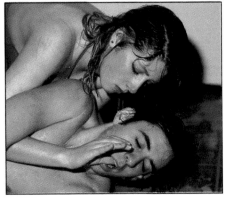

Drowning

When trying to rescue someone from drowning, remember to follow these essential points for rescue breathing.

DON'T try to drain water or fluid from the lungs of a drowning victim. The victim needs oxygen, and air will bubble through liquid in the windpipe.

DON'T worry if the patient vomits, as this is quite common. Stop long enough to turn the head and clear the mouth. When the vomiting is over, you can resume rescue breathing.

DON'T try rescue breathing on a person who is breathing normally.

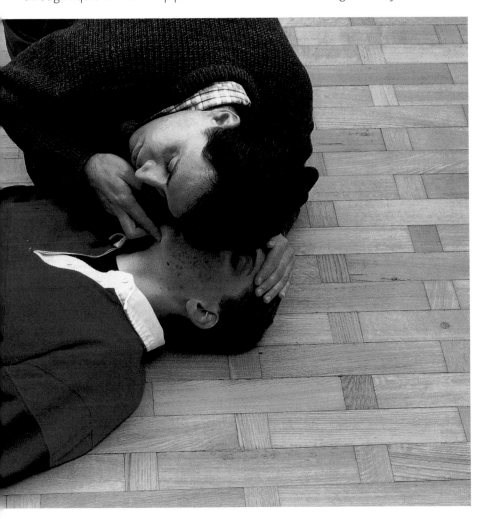

Make sure you...

DO keep fingers and hands away from the patient's lips and neck at all times, as they could obstruct breathing.

DON'T blow too hard: just raise patient's chest visibly, or you may damage the lungs.

What next?

1 Send for help as soon as possible.

2 Loosen any tight clothing. If possible, cover the patient lightly and loosely with a coat or blanket.

3 Sometimes, holding the head back may unblock the airway. The patient will probably gasp for breath.

4 Throughout first aid treatment, keep the head tilted back.

5 Check periodically to see if the patient has started to breathe naturally. If not, begin rescue breathing again, starting with four quick breaths and then single puffs. If breathing has started, keep the head back and watch carefully in case breathing stops again. Once respiration is steady, treat as if unconscious (see page 914).

6 Continue rescue breathing until breathing starts naturally or medical help arrives. Don't give up.

Always check first to see if the victim is breathing before you start rescue breathing. One way to find out is to hold a pair of glasses in front of his mouth—if the glass mists over, the victim is breathing. Cover the patient as quickly as possible with a blanket or overcoat to prevent heat loss. Covering should be loose, though, with the chest clearly visible so that you can see whether the patient is breathing.

Shock

- Shock is caused by many types of severe injury; this causes the circulation to fail, limiting the amount of oxygen carried to the body's cells
- Always tend major injuries first
- Minimize shock by laying the patient down at the site of the accident, keeping his or her head low and legs raised
- Loosen tight clothing and keep lightly covered

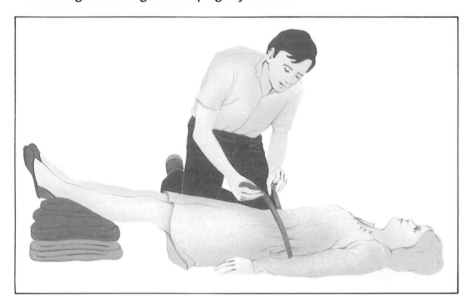

1 *Stop any bleeding (see page 894). Lie the patient down with head low and legs raised about 8–12 in. (20–30 cm). Reduce movement.*

2 *Loosen tight clothing such as belts and collars. Cover wounds with clean, dry material (see page 916). Check that the patient is comfortable.*

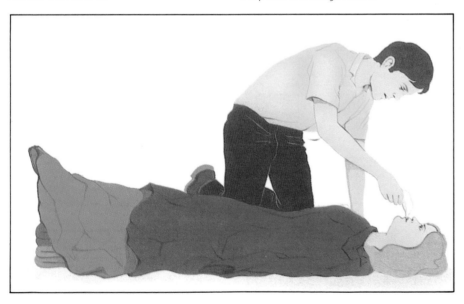

3 *Cover patient loosely with coats or blankets. Do not overheat. Reassure the patient about what you are doing.*

4 *If the patient is thirsty, soak a piece of clean cloth in water and let him or her suck it. Stay until help comes.*

Take note

- Shock is caused by a marked loss of body fluid. This may be caused by internal or external bleeding, or by blood plasma loss as a result of a serious burn.

- Body fluid loss causes the heart to beat faster and weaker. Blood pressure falls. As a consequence, the entire body receives inadequate supplies of oxygen.

- First aid should be given to prevent shock even if an accident victim looks and feels normal. Treat for breathing, bleeding, burns, and fractures first.

- A badly shocked victim may be pale, bluish, cold, and sweaty and will be mentally slow. Breathing will be shallow, and the pulse will be fast and feeble.

What next?

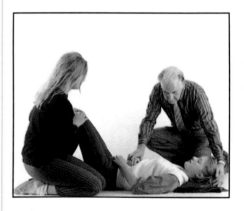

1 Keep a careful watch on the patient. Make sure that he or she is breathing properly, and that he or she does not start or resume bleeding and does not vomit. Cover with a blanket but do not use hot water bottles or electric blankets.

2 Do not give the victim any food, drink, or medicines. Stimulants such as alcohol and cigarettes should be strictly avoided.

3 Even if the patient seems unconscious, do not talk or whisper to bystanders. He or she may hear you and understand what is being said—the person needs reassurance, not more anxiety.

Sprains and Strains

- Let the patient rest the injured part in the most comfortable position, slightly raised if possible
- Cover the affected area with a cold compress, and reapply the compress every four hours
- Protect the area with a thick cloth pad
- Bandage from well below injured area to well above it

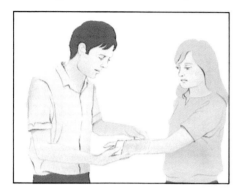

1 *A sprain involves damage to the ligaments around a joint. Apply a cold compress as soon as possible, then remove it and cover with a pad.*

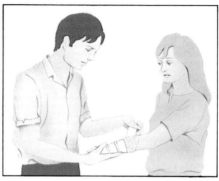

2 *Starting below the damaged joint, firmly wrap a bandage around it. Leave strips of padding visible. Immobilize the area by placing the arm in a sling.*

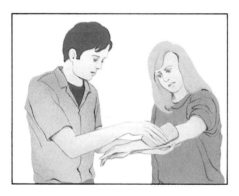

3 *Cover the strain injury with a cold compress and reapply every 4 hours for a day, then remove it. Make a thick pad.*

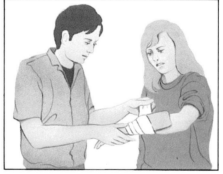

4 *Wrap an elastic bandage around the injured area firmly, but not tightly, and cover the padding.*

Take note

- In both strains and sprains, the muscle or ligament has been overstretched by a powerful movement. Small blood vessels can be torn and a bruise forms. The area will be bruised, painful, and swollen.

- Swelling can be minimized by cooling the area with a cold compress. This should be applied within half an hour of the injury. After this, there will be swelling, and no amount of cooling will help reduce it.

- To make a cold compress, soak a thick cloth in cold water. Wring it out so it is just moist. Place it on the sore area for about half an hour; moisten if it begins to warm up or dry out.

- If you think there is a chance that the patient has fractured a bone, treat accordingly (see page 904). Doctors often do exactly this until they can see the results of an X ray.

What next?

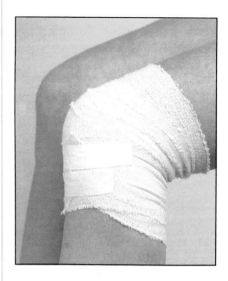

1 A strain or sprain needs rest and support in the form of a firm bandage. An elastic bandage is best, but do not put it on so tightly that it damages the underlying nerves and blood vessels. A thick pad helps to protect the area from constriction. Ask the patient to tell you if any part of the affected limb becomes cold, numb, or puffy. The bandage may be too tight.

2 If pain is severe, but there is clearly no other injury, the patient can take aspirin or acetaminophen. But never take a chance; if the pain seems too severe and you have the slightest doubt about a possible fracture, see a doctor urgently.

3 If a body part is not working properly, if there is great pain, if the injured area is misshapen in any way, or if it appears that the circulation beyond the injury has been impaired, get medical help immediately.

4 Sprains and strains are often more of a problem than people realize. Bandaging supports the limb and reduces pain, but movement is still very limited. Several days may go by before normal activity can be resumed. Check with your doctor before you do anything strenuous. A delay in repairing joints and muscles may lead to permanent damage.

Traffic Accidents

- Search the area for any people thrown clear of the vehicles
- Establish an order for treatment priority among the victims
- Treat patients for breathing problems, bleeding, and unconsciousness
- Send for emergency services, giving thorough details of the accident

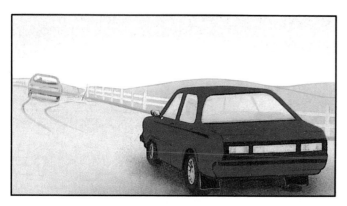

1 *If you notice that an automobile has had some kind of accident, stop a short distance away and park your vehicle safely off the road.*

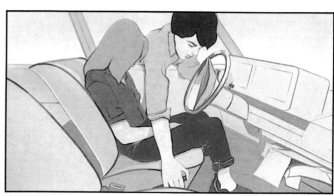

2 *Extinguish any fire if smoke is coming from vehicles, but leave victims in position unless fire is a risk. Prevent further damage by immobilizing vehicles.*

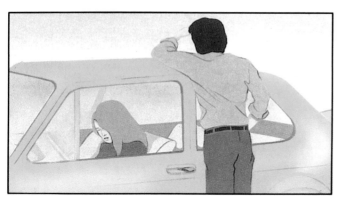

3 *Look for victims who have been thrown clear of vehicles, into ditches or over hedges. Check all the victims and make a decision whom to treat first.*

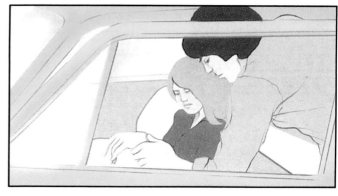

4 *Treat victims in order of priority. Deal with breathing problems, bleeding, and unconsciousness in that order. Move victims as little as possible.*

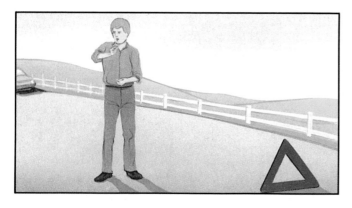

5 *Set up a warning sign in a safe place. Onlookers can direct traffic during the emergency.*

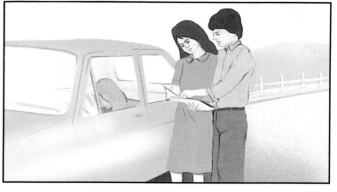

6 *Send the first available person to call emergency services, giving location, number of cars and injured, and injuries.*

Always be prepared

All drivers should carry a first aid kit in the car. Many accident victims who die before reaching the hospital could have been saved if simple first aid measures had been taken promptly.

A car first aid kit should be kept in a clearly marked waterproof case, preferably in the glove compartment. The kit should include the following:

- packs of gauze and cotton
- 2- and 3-in. (5- and 7.5-cm) bandages
- medium and large sterile dressings
- a large flashlight
- a large pair of scissors

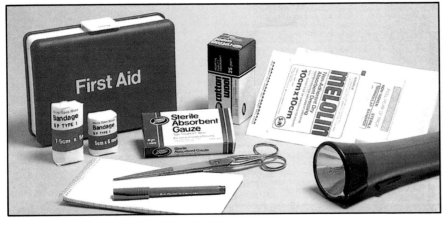

Make sure you...

DO make sure that there are no more accident victims. Alert passing traffic that an accident has happened.

DO check that the vehicles are safe. Switch off the ignition, apply brakes.

DO use any available material, such as car blankets or coats, to keep the victims warm.

DON'T move accident victims from vehicles unless there is a danger of fire, explosion, or drowning; you may make injuries worse. The rescue vehicles have special tools to cut people out of wrecked cars.

DON'T let anyone smoke anywhere near the location of the accident—leaking gasoline may catch fire.

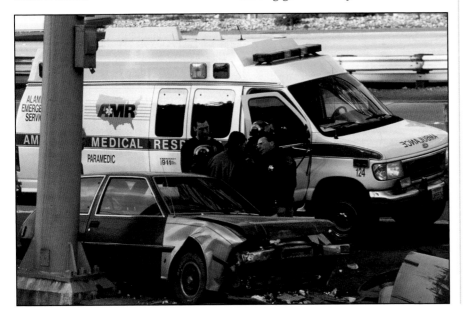

What next?

1 While you are waiting for the emergency services, try to discourage other motorists and passersby from hanging around unless they can offer expert help.

2 Keep area between your car and the accident clear at all times so that emergency services will be able to stop safely near the accident.

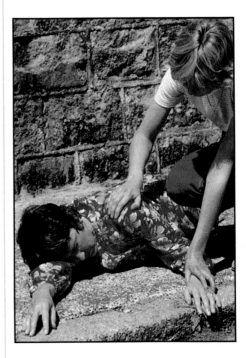

3 Stay with the victims until the ambulances arrive. Watch them carefully to make sure that breathing does not stop, bleeding does not resume, and no one loses consciousness. Try to appear confident and be reassuring—let them know that help is on the way.

4 While you are waiting for help to arrive, use any spare time to gather information to help the emergency services. Collect a list of names and addresses from the least injured victims and make a note of the vehicle license plates. Give this information to the police or paramedics when they arrive. Give a thorough account of any first aid measures that you have taken.

Unconsciousness

- **If the patient is not breathing, begin rescue breathing immediately**
- **Clear the patient's mouth**
- **Control any bleeding, check for other wounds and for possible fractures**
- **If it is safe, move the patient into recovery position and get help**

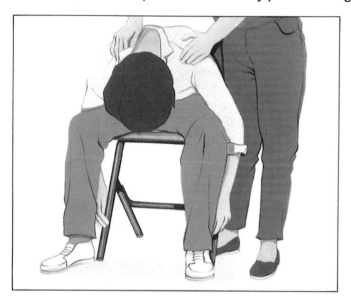

1 *If a person who is sitting down feels faint and it is impossible for him or her to lie down, tell him or her to bend all the way forward, with the head low between the knees. The victim should try to relax completely. Stay next to the person to hold him or her in case of loss of consciousness.*

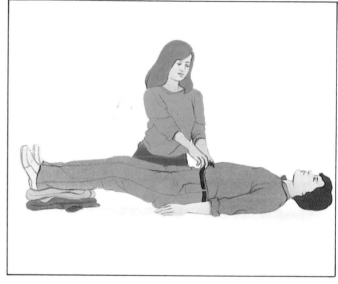

2 *Whenever possible, lie the patient down, head low and legs raised. Loosen tight clothing at the neck, chest, and waist. If the patient is conscious, tell him or her to take deep, slow breaths. When recovered, give cool water to drink. Advise the patient to remain still for five minutes before sitting up slowly.*

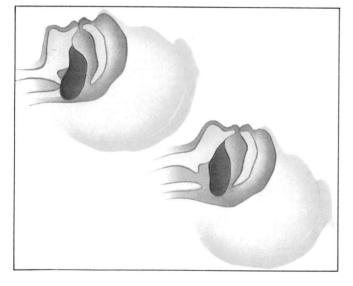

1 *When a person is unconscious, the tongue is likely to flop backward and obstruct the opening of the windpipe. Bend the head right back; the tongue will then be carried up with the jaw and the airway will open. Do this without twisting the neck. If necessary, perform rescue breathing.*

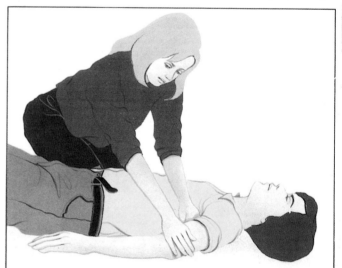

2 *Stop bleeding (see page 894) and dress wounds (see page 916). Check for fractures. Feel firmly but gently, with hands flat, from one end of the body to the other, taking note of any swelling. If you suspect a fracture, do not move the patient. Put him or her in the recovery position and cover with a blanket.*

Make sure you...

DO remember to check the patient's breathing before you do anything else. If he or she is lying face up, the tongue may be obstructing the airway. This must be treated as an emergency.

DO remove anything, such as a pillow, from under the patient's head if he or she is breathing with difficulty.

DO follow the routine to safeguard breathing, stop bleeding, and protect against further harm before moving the patient into the recovery position.

DON'T twist or turn the neck when moving the head, in case there has been some injury to the upper part of the spinal column.

DON'T try to make the unconscious person drink. The fluid would run into the windpipe. Even if he or she responds vaguely to touch and speech, the ability to swallow may be impaired.

CPR (cardiopulmonary resuscitation)

Cardiopulmonary arrest means that there is no breathing or heartbeat. CPR is a mixture of rescue breathing and chest compressions. It attempts to provide oxygen to the patient's lungs and to keep the heart beating so that oxygenated blood can circulate around the body. For CPR, carry out the following steps.
• First, check that the victim's airway is not blocked. If you think it is, do first aid for choking (see page 898), then open airway–lift up the chin by placing your hand on the victim's forehead, put two fingers of the other hand under the bony part of the victim's chin and tilt the head back.
• Ascertain if the person is breathing by looking and listening. Chest movement alone does not mean that someone is breathing. If the victim is not breathing, begin rescue breathing (see page 908). Check to see if the victim's chest rises. If it does not, the airway may be blocked.
• Check whether there is a pulse. With the victim's head tilted, check the carotid pulse in the neck for 5–10 seconds. Place two fingers in the groove between the voice box and the muscle at the side of the neck.

Don't use your thumb because you will feel your own pulse. If the victim is breathing and has a pulse, keep monitoring both, and check for other injuries. If the person is not breathing and there is no pulse (i.e., the patient's heart is not beating), start CPR. Meanwhile, get someone else to call for help, or if you are alone, perform CPR for one minute, then call emergency services. To position your hands for CPR, find notch where the ribs meet the breastbone in the center of the chest. Place middle finger on the notch and index finger next to it. Place heel of other hand next to and above index finger. Remove fingers from notch and place the heel of this hand over the heel of the other hand. At the rate of 80 to 100 per minute, give 15 chest compressions, using the weight of your body to compress the breastbone by about 2 in. (5 cm). Open the airway and give two more breaths; check if the chest rises. Continue this sequence of 15 compressions and 2 breaths for 4 cycles. If there is a pulse and breathing, stop CPR. If there is a pulse but no breathing, continue rescue breathing. If there is no breathing and no pulse, repeat CPR.

Take note

• Examine the patient to see if he or she is breathing. If not, begin rescue breathing immediately (see page 908).

• Look for any severe bleeding. Control it at once (see page 894).

• Check for any other wounds. Cover them at once with a dressing (you may have to improvise one; see page 916).

• Search for possible fractures. If you suspect a fracture that would be made worse by moving the patient, do not move him or her. Remember, a fractured spine is almost impossible to detect in an unconscious patient. The patient must definitely not be moved.

• If it is safe to move the patient, turn him or her gently into the recovery position shown below.

• Get medical help immediately.

What next?

1 The cause of the patient's unconsciousness may be unknown. The doctor must be the person to diagnose and to treat. Your responsibility is to get help immediately and administer first aid, if necessary.

2 Even if there is no sign of emergency at first, watch the patient in case breathing stops and rescue breathing is needed, or he or she vomits. If this happens, clear the mouth using a curved finger.

3 If you do not know the patient and you will not harm him or her with your movements, look for any cards, bracelets, badges, or other medical alert tags. They will tell you if the patient suffers from a condition such as diabetes or epilepsy and should be handed to the doctor or paramedics.

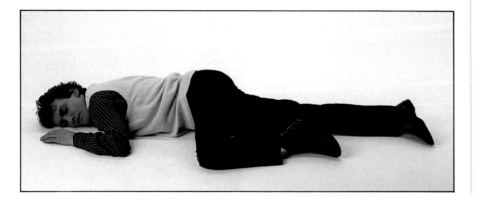

Wounds

- Wash the skin in and around the wound, moving outward from the wound
- Put gauze and then a thick pad over the wound and bandage firmly
- Keep the patient, and especially the injured part, at rest
- Reassure the patient, protect against shock and get help

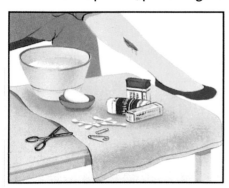
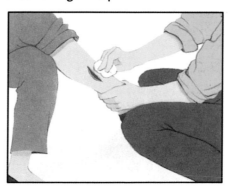
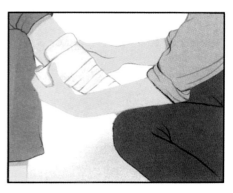

1 *To dress a wound, you need several articles from a first aid box: absorbent cotton, gauze, and bandages. You will also need mild soap and water.*

2 *Wash wound and skin around it with cotton moistened with warm water and soap; flush with water. Work outward from wound; blot dry with sterile gauze.*

3 *Put gauze over the wound, covering beyond the wound area. Place a thick pad over the gauze and bandage the dressing securely.*

Making a ring pad

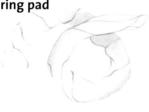

1 *Use a long, thin piece of folded cloth, or a large handkerchief. Form one end into a circle.*

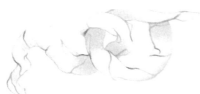

2 *Hold the circle and slip the end through the loop. Keep looping the long, free end around the circle.*

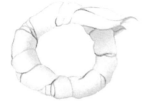

3 *When the cloth has been totally used up, you will have a firm, thick ring to protect a wound.*

Objects in wounds

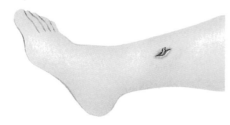

1 *If an object is lying on the surface of a wound, brush it away with a clean piece of gauze. However, if an object has become embedded, leave it undisturbed. Let trained medical personnel remove it.*

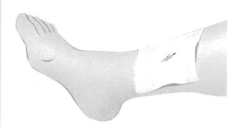

2 *Carefully cover the wound with a piece of sterile gauze big enough to extend well beyond the area of the wound itself. If the gauze is too small, it may slip and expose part of the wound.*

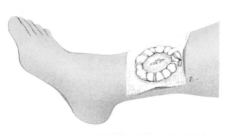

3 *Make a ring pad from a large handkerchief or a small towel. Place it around the object in the wound. This will prevent the object from being further pressed into the wound by any bandage you put over it. Once the wound is bandaged, seek expert medical help.*

Take note

• Sit or lie the patient down.

• Protect the wound temporarily with the cleanest cover you can find. Wash your hands and collect the material needed: soap, water, cotton balls, gauze, bandages (or their improvised substitutes). Place them nearby on a clean surface.

• Wash the wound and the skin around it. Use cotton moistened with water and mild soap; follow with clear water. Use a clean cotton ball for each separate stroke, moving outward from the wound.

• Put gauze over the wound; make sure it is large enough to extend well beyond the injury and over the cleaned skin.

• On top of the gauze, gently place a thick pad of absorbent cotton.

• Bandage firmly, but not tightly.

• Keep the injured part at rest.

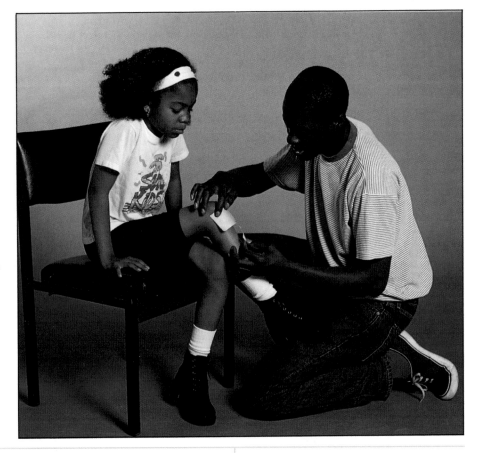

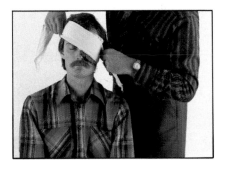

Dressings

• Convenient, ready-made, all-in-one dressings come with the gauze and pad attached to the bandage.

• Adhesive bandages come in continuous strips and can be cut to size to dress small, superficial wounds.

• An improvised gauze dressing can be made from clean materials such as a handkerchief, towel, or pillowcase. One or two folded handkerchiefs will serve as a pad. Cloths can be used as bandages.

Dressing an eye wound

For an eye wound, bandage or tape a large soft clean pad over the whole eye, without putting any pressure on it. If it hurts the patient to move his eye, cover both eyes, as the two automatically move together. Seek medical help—trying to remove foreign bodies may do more damage than good.

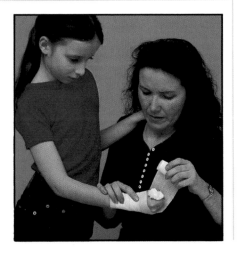

What next?

1 The slight bleeding of most wounds is soon brought under control by the pressure of ordinary bandages. (If bleeding is severe, see page 894.)

2 If possible, wash your hands or wear sterile gloves before dealing with the victim's wound. The aim of first aid in the case of wounds is to protect the part from becoming infected and damaged further. First aid should be limited to cleaning around the wound, if circumstances permit, and to covering it.

3 Do not use antiseptic or antibiotic lotions and creams without a prescription. They may interfere with healing.

4 With any wound, there is the risk of tetanus. The deeper the cut, the higher the risk. Even if the patient has been immunized against tetanus, he should still see a doctor.

Landmarks in Health and Medicine

The remains of prehistoric people show they practiced medicine thousands of years ago. They believed that anything unexplained was the work of good or evil spirits, and early medicine was considered a part of magic. To prevent illnesses, they carried charms or magical objects. To cure diseases, they made offerings to their gods or cast spells. The life expectancy of prehistoric man was about 29 years; by the end of the nineteenth century, it was 50 years. In the twenty-first century, due to improvements in sanitation and nutrition, it is 20 to 30 years longer. Vaccination programs and antibiotics prevent millions of deaths each year. However, lifestyle factors, accidents, and aging bring a new set of health problems.

Ancient medicine

An early cure for insanity
Around 8000 B.C.E., some people practiced trepanning, cutting holes in the skull. They did this to release the spirits that they suspected were causing madness or epilepsy.

Medical prescriptions on clay and papyrus
The earliest known writing about medicine dates from around 3500 B.C.E. A woman physician in Mesopotamia left a collection of prescriptions on clay tablets. Around the same time, Egyptian doctors made the first scientific study of the human body and its ailments.

A doctor declared a god
The first physician was Imhotep, who was in the service of Pharaoh Zoser of Egypt around 2650 B.C.E. He was chief minister to the pharaoh and also an architect, designing the first pyramid. He is the only doctor to have been declared a god.

Earliest false teeth
In the 700s B.C.E., the Etruscans in northern Italy made the earliest known false teeth from bone or ivory.

Hippocrates and his oath
About 400 B.C.E., the Greek physician Hippocrates established the pattern for modern medicine with case histories and bedside observations. He established a code of conduct for doctors, which is now enshrined in the Hippocratic Oath. This states that the patient's welfare is a doctor's main concern. The Romans added to medical knowledge, too. After that came a period of history called the Dark Ages, when almost no advances in scientific knowledge were made.

100–1499 C.E.

Galen discovers blood in arteries
The writings of the Greek physician Galen, who lived from 130–200 mainly in Rome, were standard texts for centuries. Galen discovered that the arteries contain blood.

First medical textbooks
Luckily, many Greek medical texts were preserved by being translated into Arabic. In about 1020, Avicenna, a Persian physician and philosopher, wrote a Canon of Medicine. It was used as a medical textbook for more than 600 years. Around 925, the Persian physician Rhazes (Abu Bakr Muhammad ibn Zakariyya) compiled a Greco-Arabic encyclopedia of medicine, entitled *Kitab al-Hami*. The first major medical school in Europe was founded in 1000 at Salerno, Italy.

Early plastic surgery
About 1200, Hindu doctors in India began using plastic surgery to repair the noses of people who had had them cut off as a punishment for committing adultery.

Chinese eyeglasses and toothbrushes
The Chinese also had a flourishing medical tradition. The Venetian traveler Marco Polo reported that he saw Chinese people wearing glasses in 1275. This is the earliest mention of eyeglasses, and in 1498, a Chinese encyclopedia described the modern type of toothbrush.

1500–1699

First cesarean birth in Europe
The Renaissance period in Europe saw a revival of interest in medicine. This period was a rebirth of learning after the Dark Ages. However, one important medical event of this time was not associated with scholarship. The operation of cesarean section, by which a baby is delivered through a surgical incision in the abdomen, had been known since Roman times, when it was used to deliver babies from dead or dying mothers. In 1500, Jacob Nüfer from Sigershauffen, Switzerland, performed the first known cesarean section in Europe on his wife, after doctors were unable to help her. She lived and had five more children.

Artificial limbs for soldiers
Surgeons became more skilled, though operations were carried out without anesthetics. The greatest surgeon of the 1500s was Ambroise Paré, a French military surgeon. He revolutionized wound treatment and in 1540 made moving artificial limbs for wounded soldiers to wear.

Discoveries about anatomy and circulation
A landmark in medicine came in 1543 when the Flemish anatomist Andreas Vesalius published his book *On the Fabric of the Human Body*. It was the first accurate description of

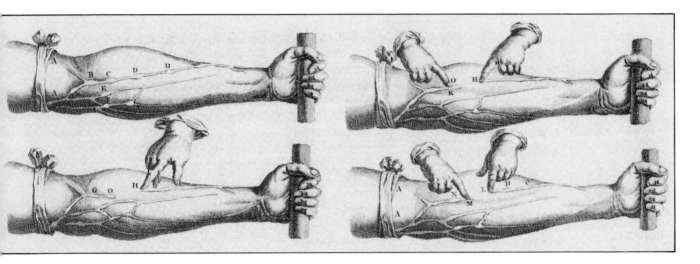

William Harvey illustrated how blood in the arm flows continuously in one direction, controlled by valves in the veins (above).

the body. Another landmark was achieved in 1628 when the English physician William Harvey published *De motu cordis*, in which he described for the first time the circulation of the blood around the body. Before that, doctors thought blood ebbed and flowed like the tide.

Wheelchairs
Modern medicine began in the 1800s, but there were a few more highlights in the 1600s and 1700s. In 1650, Stephen Farfler, a physically disabled man from Nuremberg, Germany, made a crank-driven three-wheeled chair to take him to church.

Smallpox inoculation
In 1668, a Welsh girl, 12-year-old Margaret Brown, became the first person in Europe to be inoculated against smallpox with material from smallpox blisters. This was a forerunner of vaccination.

The first microscope
Research and understanding took a great leap forward in the 1670s. Antony van Leewenhoek, who was a Dutch shopkeeper, built the first microscope and was the first person to describe bacteria, capillaries, and spermatozoa.

By the late nineteenth century, the stethoscope was widely used when examining patients (right).

First medical journal
The first medical journal was published in 1671. It was the *Acta* of the Royal Medical and Philosophical Society of Copenhagen, Denmark.

1700–1849

Ben Franklin's bifocals
American doctors depended on Europe for their training for years. In 1765, the first medical school in North America was established at the University of Pennsylvania. In 1784, Benjamin Franklin invented bifocal lenses for glasses.

Origins of vaccination
Today, we take preventive medicine for granted, but it really dates from 1796, the year the British physician Edward Jenner, popularizer of vaccination, inoculated a patient to induce cowpox as a preventive against smallpox.

Plastic surgery in the West
Plastic surgery was introduced into Western medicine in 1814. The English surgeon Joseph Carpus, who had seen the Hindu doctors' skill in this form of operation, restored the nose of an army officer at York Hospital, Chelsea, London.

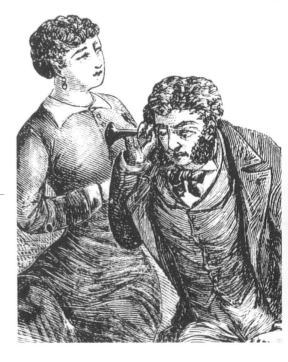

Invention of the stethoscope
Modern doctors use a stethoscope to help them examine patients. This medical tool was invented in 1815 by a French physician René Laënnec.

First successful blood transfusion
Another familiar technique is that of blood transfusion. For centuries, it was common practice to take blood from patients to reduce their fever. However, during the 1700s, several doctors tried to transfuse blood from animals to people, or from one person to another. The results were poor, because the body rejected

the alien blood. In 1825, the first successful human blood transfusion was performed by Dr. James Blundell in London, but the operation remained risky for many years.

Barbers as surgeons

Surgeons were growing more skilled as time went on, but surgery as a whole was risky. The surgeons were originally barbers who did operations as a sideline, and even after they became properly trained members of the medical profession, surgery was a painful and hazardous process. It was carried out in dirty conditions, using instruments that were not sterilized. Surgeons wore their oldest garments when operating. These clothes were often caked with blood from earlier operations, and a large number of patients died from infections.

Early painkillers

Surgeons had to work fast when operating, not only because of the risk of shock to the patients but also to reduce the loss of blood and pain experienced during the operation. There was some knowledge of painkilling drugs; the Chinese surgeon Hua T'o, who lived from 115 to 205 C.E., used a powder dissolved in wine that produced a form of anesthesia. Surgeons used opium, cannabis, mandrake, and henbane to reduce pain, or gave patients large quantities of alcohol. Even so, many operations were carried out without any form of painkillers, particularly on the battlefield.

Laughing gas

In 1799, British scientist Humphry Davy found that so-called laughing gas, or nitrous oxide, had anesthetic properties. No one acted on this discovery until 1844, when Horace Wells, a dentist from Hartford, Conn., saw that a man who hurt his leg during a demonstration of laughing gas felt no pain. The next day, he persuaded a fellow dentist to give him laughing gas while he pulled a tooth, and he also felt no pain.

Ether and chloroform

Two years earlier, in 1842, William Clarke, an American medical student, used ether as an anesthetic while a friend was having a tooth extracted. Later the same year, Crawford W. Long, a physician from Athens, Georgia, was the first doctor to use ether for surgery. Ether did not come into general use until 1846, when dentist William T. G. Morton demonstrated its use at Massachusetts General Hospital in Boston. Ether proved to be a safe anesthetic, and its use enabled surgeons to perform more complex operations. In 1847, Sir James Young Simpson, a Scottish obstetrician, first used chloroform to relieve the pain of childbirth.

Problem of infection

In 1846, Ignaz Semmelweis, who was a Hungarian obstetrician, discovered that infection from surgeons' hands was a major cause of death to women in childbirth. This pointed the way to future developments.

First woman doctor in America

In 1847, the American Medical Association was founded in Philadelphia. Two years later came another landmark in American medicine when Elizabeth Blackwell became the first woman to receive an M.D. degree in North America.

1850–1899

Hypodermic syringe

Charles Gabriel Pravaz, a physician who lived in Lyon, France, invented the hypodermic syringe in 1853. The hollow needle for injections had been invented back in 1844 by Francis Rynd, an Irish physician. These inventions made it possible to administer drugs under the skin.

Lister and antiseptics

The greatest steps in safe surgery came after the French chemist Louis Pasteur discovered in 1864 that fermentation in beer, milk, and wine is caused by microorganisms. This made the English surgeon Joseph Lister realize that microbes were the cause of infection in wounds. He decided that the best way of combating the microbes was to use chemicals to kill them. In 1865, he performed the first operation under antiseptic conditions at Glasgow Royal Infirmary, using carbolic acid.

A dilute solution of the acid was sprayed over everything in the operating room—instruments, towels, dressings, clothing, even the patient and the staff. There was no infection of the wound, but over a period of time, nurses and surgeons started to suffer from carbolic acid poisoning.

Sterilization of instruments

German surgeon Ernst von Bergman introduced the idea of asepsis— killing bacteria to prevent them from entering the operating room at all. In 1886, he began sterilizing instruments and dressings by steam heat, and five years later made sure that everything connected with the operating room was sterilized, too.

First electric dental drill

George F. Green from Kalamazoo, Mich. invented the first electric dental drill in 1875. A mechanical drill had been invented in 1863 by a British dentist, George Fellows Harrington.

Cause of TB discovered

Pasteur's work in microbiology was continued by, among others, the German bacteriologist Robert Koch. In 1882, Koch isolated the bacillus that causes tuberculosis.

Vaccines for rabies and plague

In 1882, Louis Pasteur began his studies into the dreaded and fatal disease of rabies. In 1885, he produced a vaccine to protect animals and people against it and successfully vaccinated Joseph Meister, a nine-year-old boy. In 1894, the Swiss bacteriologist Alexandre Yersin, who was serving as a medical officer in the French colonial service, identified the bacillus that causes bubonic plague. He then made an effective vaccine against it. His work helped to control epidemics of the plague and other diseases in the French colonies in Southeast Asia.

The first incubator
Deaths of children, particularly premature babies, were very common. A major step forward in keeping premature babies alive was taken in 1891 when the first incubator for babies was introduced by Dr. Alexandre Lion from Nice, France.

Discovery of X rays
The most important element in the treatment of illness is diagnosis—deciding what is actually wrong with a patient.

One of the greatest aids to diagnosis came in 1895. Wilhelm Roentgen, a German physicist who was a professor in Würzburg, Germany, discovered X rays. The first clinical X-ray photograph was taken in Vienna that year.

Doctors hailed this new technique with delight, and within a few months X rays were being used in many countries to examine broken bones. The modern X-ray tube was devised by an American physicist, William D. Coolidge, in 1913.

At first, however, ordinary people were suspicious of this unknown test. For a while, there was a trade in X-ray–proof undergarments for ladies who were fearful of what others might see!

Value of aspirin
One of the most important medical developments in the nineteenth century came in 1899 when aspirin was discovered.

The value of aspirin (acetylsalicylic acid) as a drug was first recognized by a German scientist, Heinrich Dreser. Aspirin is one of the most commonly used modern drugs. It is prescribed to relieve pain, especially in cases of arthritis and headaches, and to reduce both fever and

inflammation. In recent years, doctors have begun prescribing small, regular doses of aspirin to prevent blood clots, which cause strokes and heart attacks in those people who are at risk.

1900–1949

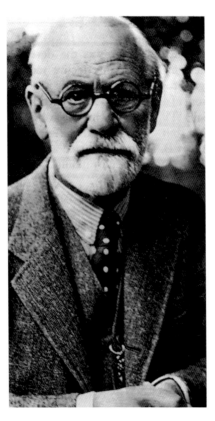

Sigmund Freud used people's dreams and unconscious thoughts to help him treat mental illness.

Freud and psychoanalysis
During the early 1900s, the Austrian neurologist Sigmund Freud evolved the technique of psychoanalysis for treating mental illness.

Blood groups and blood typing
In 1901, the Austrian-American pathologist Karl Landsteiner classified the A-B-O blood types. As a result, six years later, blood transfusion became safe when the practice of blood typing—matching

a patient's blood to the donor blood—was introduced. A further advance came in 1940. Landsteiner and others discovered the rhesus factor in blood types, which caused many illnesses in newborn babies.

Detecting heart disease
A valuable aid to diagnosis was created in 1903. Dutch physiologist Willem Einthoven made the first clinical use of the electrocardiograph for detecting heart disorders at Leyden Hospital in the Netherlands. From 1909, the electrocardiograph was used in the United States.

Discovery of vitamins
Diet has always been an important factor in good health. In 1906, British biochemist Frederick Hopkins announced the important discovery of the role of vitamins in diet and in this way explained why certain foods were necessary for the maintenance of good health.

Insulin for diabetes
Diabetes is a disease that affects about 11 million Americans. Its treatment was revolutionized after 1921, when Canadian physician Frederick Banting, working with physiologist Charles Best and John J. R. Macleod, isolated insulin, a substance involved in the disease. Regular injections of insulin have saved the lives of millions of people.

The iron lung
Paralysis of the muscles used in breathing, often a side effect of poliomyelitis, frequently caused death. Treatment became more effective after Philip Drinker and Louis A. Shaw of Harvard School of Public Health invented the iron lung, or respirator, in 1928. This device saved many lives in the United States during the polio epidemics of the 1950s.

EEG for brain disorders
Just as the electrocardiograph helped in the diagnosis of heart disease, so the invention of the

electroencephalograph (EEG) in 1934 by the British neurophysiologist Edgar D. Adrian helped with the diagnosis of brain disorders.

First antihistamines

In 1937, hay fever sufferers received relief when the Italian chemist Daniel Bovet produced the first antihistamine drug. Antihistamines came into general use in 1942.

Chemotherapy

Perhaps the most significant advance is the development of chemotherapy to treat diseases such as cancer and leukemia. It works by directing chemicals against specific organisms or abnormal cells.

Sulfa drugs

The first drugs used to fight bacteria were the sulfonamides, discovered by the German biochemist Gerhard Domagk in 1932. They are still in use, but they can have bad side effects.

Development of antibiotics

The French-born American microbiologist René Dubos developed the first antibiotic in clinical use, gramicidin, in 1939. It was soon followed by many other antibiotics. The most important of these antibiotics is penicillin, which was discovered in 1928 by a British bacteriologist, Alexander Fleming. British researchers Howard Florey and Ernst Chain made it widely available. American drug companies mass-produced penicillin during World War II, in which it saved many lives. Another important antibiotic is streptomycin, the first effective treatment for TB. It was discovered in 1943 by Russian-born U.S. microbiologist Selman Waksman.

First artificial kidney

Kidney disease, especially kidney failure, was fatal until Dutch scientist Willem Kolff built an artificial kidney. He treated his first patient with it in 1943, in Holland. In 1950, he moved to the U.S. to develop it further.

1950–2000

Polio vaccine

In 1953, Jonas Salk, an American researcher, developed an effective vaccine against poliomyelitis. The Salk vaccine is given as a shot, but in 1960 another American, Albert B. Sabin, developed a vaccine that can be taken by mouth. Polio was eventually eradicated in 1994.

First successful kidney transplant

The first successful kidney transplant was performed by Joseph Murray, an American surgeon at the Peter Bent Brigham Hospital in Boston, Mass., in 1954. This was between identical twins, who shared tissue types. Other transplants failed because the body's immune system rejected the implanted organ. The development of immunosuppressive drugs has led to a great many successful transplants, notably of the kidney, liver, and heart.

First heart transplant

The first human heart transplant was performed in 1967 by Dr. Christiaan Barnard, a South African surgeon. The patient was Louis Washansky, a wholesale grocer, and he survived for 18 days. Heart transplant patients today have a survival expectancy of several years.

First artificial heart

Barnard's work was made possible by the development of open-heart surgery, first successfully performed in 1962 by American surgeon F. John Lewis. In 1982, the first implantation of an artificial heart was carried out in the United States.

Contraceptive pill

In 1956, Dr. Gregory Pincus of Shrewsbury, Mass., developed an oral contraceptive, using synthetic hormones.

Medicaid and Medicare

In 1965, the United States launched the Medicaid and Medicare programs, providing medical care for people who cannot afford to pay for it, and health and hospital insurance for people over 65 and some disabled people.

Smallpox vaccination

A smallpox eradication program was started in 1967. It proved to be very successful and the world was officially declared free from smallpox in December 1979.

Screening program

In 1970, screening for cervical cancer reduced the cases of the disease by 70 percent.

First test tube baby

In 1978 came the birth of the first test tube baby, Louise Brown. The technique was pioneered by the English surgeon Patrick Steptoe.

Arrival of AIDS

In 1979 came the first reported cases of AIDS (Acquired Immune Deficiency Syndrome), a new disease that has caused widespread anxiety and illness worldwide. Advances in drug treatment have meant that the virus can be suppressed, although new drug-resistant strains are appearing, and the search for a preventive vaccine continues. In 1981, safe sex guidelines were introduced.

Human genome project

In the 1990s, a huge research project was started to produce the entire gene map of all the chromosomes that contain the information needed to make a human being, and also to map out the genes that predispose a person to certain diseases. For example, using molecular biology and molecular genetics, scientists can map out the links between chromosomes, the genes within them, and diseases such as cancer.

Designer babies

In this controversial practice, couples genetically engineer a baby with desired traits. This procedure happens only rarely and is strictly controlled.

Health Heroes

Addison, Thomas (1793–1860), was a British doctor who first identified Addison's disease. This disease affects the adrenal glands. It makes the sufferer very weak and turns the skin bluish-brown. The disease was considered incurable, but it can now be treated with drugs.

Apgar, Virginia (1909–1974), an American doctor, introduced a system for deciding how healthy a newborn baby is. The Apgar Score, as it is called, gives points for the condition of parts of the body, such as the heart and muscles. The system is widely used in hospitals.

Avicenna (980–1047) was a Persian scientist and one of the greatest scholars of the Middle Ages. He studied alchemy, astronomy, mathematics, philosophy, physics, and, above all, medicine. He wrote many books. The most famous is his *Canon of Medicine*, an encyclopedia of about a million words, which covered all the medical knowledge of that particular time.

Banting, Frederick Grant (1891–1941), a Canadian doctor, helped to discover insulin, which is the substance used for treating diabetes. Banting worked as an orthopedic surgeon but spent all his spare time in a laboratory at Toronto University working with Professor J. J. R. Macleod and a student, Charles Herbert Best. Banting and Macleod were awarded a Nobel prize in 1923 for their work on insulin. Banting shared his prize money with Best. Banting continued research until World War II, when he was killed in an airplane crash.

Barton, Clara (1821–1912), founded the American Red Cross. After many years as a schoolteacher, and later a clerk, she nursed wounded men during the Civil War and took relief supplies to them on the battlefields. In 1869, she went to Europe for a vacation, but soon became involved in nursing the wounded in the Franco-Prussian War of 1870–1871. She worked with the International Red Cross and, on her return, she campaigned to have the United States join the Red Cross.

Becquerel, Antoine Henri (1852–1908), a French physicist, shared the 1903 Nobel prize in physics with Pierre and Marie Curie for discovering radioactivity. He suggested the possibility of radiation therapy, now widely used for treating disease.

Billroth, Christian Albert Theodor (1829–1894), a German surgeon, founded the modern techniques of abdominal surgery. He also discovered that bacteria cause infection in wounds. He was the first surgeon to remove the larynx from a patient with cancer.

Blackwell was the name of two sisters who were pioneer women in medicine. They were born in England and emigrated to the United States when they were children.

Elizabeth (1821–1910) became a schoolteacher but wanted to study medicine. Several medical schools rejected her, but eventually she was accepted by Geneva College of Medicine, now part of New York State University. She qualified in 1849 and became the first woman to qualify as a physician. She then studied in London and Paris, where she lost the sight of one eye due to an infection. On her return to the United States, she founded the New York Infirmary for Women and Children. She later settled in England.

Emily (1826–1910) was rejected by 11 medical schools and expelled by a twelfth, but finally qualified in 1854. She joined her sister at the New York Infirmary and became dean of the Women's Medical College there.

Bruce, David (1855–1931), an Australian-born Scottish doctor, identified the cause of the disease Malta fever, or undulant fever. Bruce found the disease was due to a bacterium, which is named *Brucella melitensis* for him. The disease is now called brucellosis.

Carrel, Alexis (1873–1944), was a pioneer in transplant surgery. He developed a method of suturing (sewing up) blood vessels, which won him a Nobel prize in 1912. French born, he spent more than 30 years at the Rockefeller Institute in New York, returning to France in 1939.

Cavell, Edith (1865–1915), a British nurse, ran a Red Cross hospital in Brussels, Belgium, during World War I. After the Germans occupied Brussels, she helped about 200 Allied soldiers to escape. For this, she was tried and shot by the Germans.

Curie was the name of a family of scientists famous for their work on radioactivity, which made radiation treatment of disease possible. **Pierre Curie** (1859–1906) was born in Paris. He married the Polish-born **Marie Sklodowska** (1867–1934), and they worked together until he was killed in a street accident. They shared the 1903 Nobel prize with Antoine Henri Becquerel. The Curies' daughter **Irène** (1897–1956) and her husband **Frédéric Joliot-Curie** carried on the study of radiation.

Cushing, Harvey Williams (1869–1939), was a leading brain surgeon who founded the modern techniques of brain surgery. He was professor of surgery at Harvard, and his pupils carried his skills and

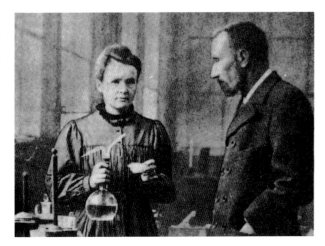

Pierre and Marie Curie shown here in the early 1900s.

knowledge all over the world. Cushing carried out many successful operations to remove brain tumors. Before his day, patients rarely survived such operations.

Dick was the name of a husband-and-wife team of physicians who discovered that scarlet fever is caused by *streptococci*. They were **George Frederick Dick** (1881–1967) and **Gladys Henry Dick** (1881–1963). They made their discovery in 1923 while working at Rush Medical College, Chicago.

A year later, they devised a test, known as the Dick test, which will show whether or not a person is susceptible to scarlet fever. They prepared drugs to prevent and cure attacks.

Dix, Dorothea Lynde (1802–1887), was responsible for changes in the way mentally ill persons are cared for in the United States.

Dorothea Dix began her career as a schoolteacher. While she was teaching Sunday school in a jail near Cambridge, Mass., she was shocked to find mentally ill people in prison with criminals.

She wrote a report about the care of mental patients, which led Massachusetts and 15 other states to build special asylums for mentally ill people. During the Civil War, Dorothea Dix was superintendent of women nurses for the Union.

Domagk, Gerhard (1895–1964), a German doctor, discovered the first of the sulfa drugs. These drugs are used to kill bacteria. In 1932, he found that a dye called Prontosil Red controlled some infections in mice. French researchers isolated the substance in the dye that controlled the infection as one of the sulfa drugs. Soon the drugs were used to fight disease in humans. Many lives were saved, including that of Domagk's own daughter. In 1939, Domagk was awarded a Nobel prize for his work, but the Nazi rulers of Germany would not let him accept it.

Drew, Charles Richard (1904–1950), pioneered blood banks. A world-renowned physician and surgeon, he organized and directed programs for the use of blood plasma in the United States and Britain during World War II. At Columbia University Hospital, New York City, he researched ways of blood preservation and he found that this could be done by just using plasma. Drew resigned from the blood plasma program when the war department ordered that blood from white and black donors was not to be mixed. He returned to a teaching post but was then fatally injured in an automobile crash. Ironically, his life might have been saved by a blood transfusion, but the hospital turned him away because he was black.

Dunant, Jean Henri (1828–1910), founded the International Red Cross. Dunant was born in Geneva, Switzerland, and became a banker. In August 1859, while war was raging between Austria and Sardinia, he visited the little village of Solferino in Lombardy, the day after a battle had been fought that left around 40,000 dead and wounded on the battlefield. Dunant led a group of volunteers to help the wounded. On his return to Switzerland, Dunant wrote a book in which he proposed that a permanent aid organization should be set up, as well as an international agreement on the treatment of people wounded in wartime. The Red Cross was founded in 1863, taking its name and emblem from the Swiss flag, but with the colors reversed. Dunant neglected his business to pursue his humanitarian ideals and spent the next 20 years of his life in poverty. In 1901, he was awarded a share in the first Nobel prize for peace.

Einthoven, Willem (1860–1927), a Dutch physiologist, discovered how to measure and record electrical impulses that the heart emits every time it beats. This electrocardiography can help doctors to detect heart disorders. Einthoven's work brought him a Nobel prize in 1924.

Fallopio, Gabriel (1523–1562), abandoned a career in the Church to become a physician. He taught anatomy at Ferrara, Pisa, and Padua, in Italy. Fallopio made many medical and anatomical discoveries, among them the tubes leading to the female uterus (womb) that are still named "fallopian" tubes for him. He was also a distinguished surgeon and botanist.

Finlay, Carlos Juan (1833–1915), discovered in 1879 that yellow fever was transmitted by the bite of a mosquito. Finlay even identified the particular species of mosquito that was responsible for carrying the disease. As a result of his work, mosquitoes in Cuba and Panama were killed off, greatly reducing yellow fever there.

Fleming, Alexander (1881–1955), discovered penicillin. He devoted his life to studying bacteria at the Royal College of Surgeons in London, where he became a professor. In 1928, he noticed that a dish containing some bacteria that he was growing had become infected with a mold, which appeared to be killing off the bacteria. He proved that the mold, which he named penicillin, not only stopped the bacteria from growing, but was also apparently harmless to human body cells. Despite this amazing discovery, Fleming did not take his research any further, but in 1945 he shared the Nobel prize for medicine with Howard Florey and Ernst Chain.

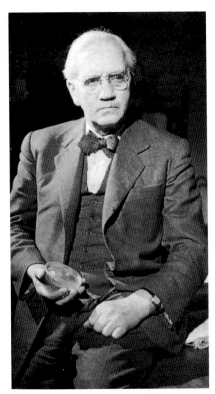

Alexander Fleming, the man who revolutionized modern medicine by discovering penicillin.

Florey, Howard Walter (1898–1968), an Australian pathologist, took Alexander Fleming's discovery of penicillin and made it into a usable drug, thereby saving thousands of lives in World War II. Florey settled in England in 1921 and worked there for the rest of his life. During World War II, he and Ernst Chain, a German-born British biochemist, began work on penicillin. They first proved that it would heal wounds and treat other illnesses, and then persuaded the big American drug companies to find ways of mass-producing the drug. For their work, Florey, Fleming, and Chain shared the 1945 Nobel prize for medicine.

Galen (c. 130–200 C.E.) was a Greek physician who is called the "father of experimental physiology." He became physician to four Roman emperors. Galen dissected many animals. He made important discoveries, which he described in some of the 400 books he wrote. Among those discoveries was that the arteries contain blood, not air as people had thought. More than 80 of Galen's books are still known. For more than 1,000 years after his death, his writings were the standard medical textbooks of Europe. Galen mixed science with religion and produced many theories that turned out to be wrong or misleading.

Galvani, Luigi (1737–1798), an Italian scientist, discovered animal electricity, that is, the way electrical currents affect the bodies of animals. Galvani noticed that the legs of a dead frog twitched when it was connected to an electrical machine, or to a lightning rod during a storm. His work provided the basis of studies of nerves in the body.

Hahnemann, Samuel (1755–1843), a German doctor who founded the method of treating disease that he called homeopathy. He had a gift for languages and supported himself through medical school by the translation of scientific books. In his day, patients were given large doses of dangerous substances such as arsenic and mercury. Hahnemann found many patients were made ill by their medicines. After much study, he developed the theory that "like cures like," provided the medicine is given in very small doses. This was the principle of homeopathy. Hahnemann tested his theories and his medicines on himself, his friends, and his students.

Hamilton, Alice (1869–1970), an American doctor, specialized in industrial diseases and their prevention. After graduating as a doctor, she spent 22 years at Hull House, Chicago, an institution set up to help new settlers in the United States. For part of that time, she was also a consultant for the U.S. Labor Department, inspecting industrial establishments and reporting on the danger of workers being poisoned. Dr. Hamilton's work led to improvements in factory conditions and in compensation for injuries at work. Later she joined the medical faculty at Harvard University, the first woman to do so.

Harvey, William (1578–1657), an English physician, discovered how the blood circulates around the body. This was to be one of the most important discoveries in medicine. Harvey studied medicine at Padua, Italy, with Hieronymus Fabricius, the distinguished Italian anatomist and surgeon, and was physician to kings James I and Charles I. In 1628, Harvey published his discoveries about the heart and how it pumps blood around the body. He retired at the age of 68 and wrote a book on the reproduction and development of animals (1651).

Hippocrates (c. 460–377 B.C.E.), a Greek physician, is regarded as the father of modern medicine. Hardly anything is known about him, except that he was born on the Greek island of Kos and traveled widely. A collection of medical works, was made about 100 years after his death. His high principles led many people to regard him as the ideal physician. Some newly qualified doctors still take the Hippocratic Oath, a promise to follow the highest standards in medicine, which is traditionally but incorrectly attributed to him. The oath declares that doctors should keep patient information confidential, and that the patient's welfare must be a doctor's main concern.

Imhotep was an Egyptian physician who lived about 4,700 years ago. He is the first medical practitioner whose name we know. He was doctor and chief minister to Pharaoh Zoser. His medical skills were so admired that, after he died, the Egyptians honored him as a god. Imhotep also designed the Step Pyramid at Saqqara as a tomb for Zoser. It is still standing.

Jenner, Edward (1749–1823), a British doctor, pioneered vaccination to protect people against smallpox. He infected his patients with a similar disease called cowpox, having been told that dairy maids who caught this disease from their cows never caught smallpox.

Keller, Helen Adams (1880–1968), the American lecturer and writer, who had lost her sight and hearing by the age of 19 months, spent her life helping the blind and the deaf-blind. At the age of 16, she learned to talk and went to college. She lectured in many countries on behalf of the blind and wrote several books.

Kenny, Elizabeth (1886–1952), developed a treatment for victims of poliomyelitis while she was working as a nurse in the Australian outback. Her unconventional muscle therapy rather than the usual immobilization with casts and splints was accepted

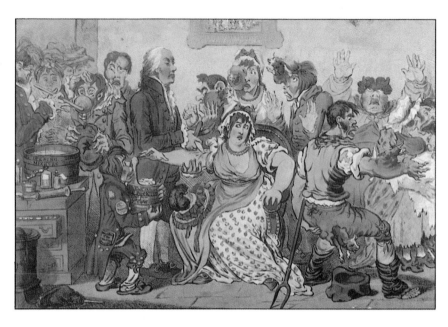

in Australia, and also in the United States, where in 1940, she established the Elizabeth Kenny Institute in Minneapolis, Minn.

Koch, Robert (1843–1910), a German doctor, won the 1905 Nobel Prize for medicine for discovering the

This early nineteenth-century cartoon makes fun of Edward Jenner's cowpox vaccination against smallpox.

Helen Keller, herself blind and deaf, became a famous author and advocate for the blind and the deaf-blind.

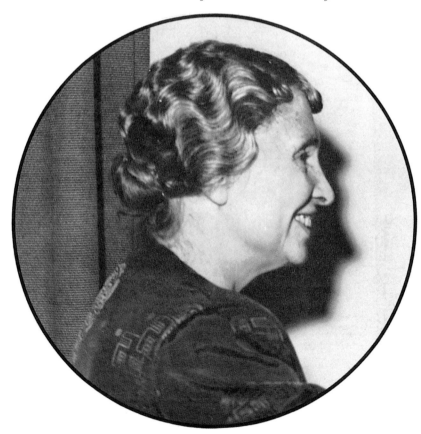

tubercle bacillus, which was found to cause tuberculosis. He is thought of as one of the leading pioneers of bacteriology as a science. Koch introduced steam sterilization and founded the Institute for Infectious Diseases in Berlin.

Laënnec, René (1781–1826), a French physician, invented the stethoscope and also the techniques of listening to and interpreting sounds in the body (auscultation). He was an expert on tuberculosis, from which, ironically, he died.

Laveran, Charles (1845–1922), a French army doctor, discovered the parasite that causes malaria while treating soldiers in Algeria. Laveran was awarded the 1907 Nobel prize for medicine.

Lister, Joseph (1827–1912), founded antiseptic surgery. Before his day, most operation wounds became infected, and half the patients died. In 1865, Lister realized that bacteria

Surgery taking place in the early days of antisepsis (below). A steam-operated carbolic spray was used to kill any germs.

caused the infection. He used carbolic sprays to kill germs in the air and insisted that surgeons used antiseptics on their hands, instruments, and dressings.

Long, Crawford Williamson (1815–1878), an American surgeon, was the first doctor to anesthetize patients with ether before surgery. He anesthetized eight patients between 1842 and the time in 1846 when William Morton, a Boston dentist, claimed to have discovered the use of ether.

Malpighi, Marcello (1628–1694), an Italian physician, discovered the red blood corpuscles and the capillaries. He became a professor at Messina, Pisa, and Bologna, and physician to the pope. He was one of the first people to use a microscope in medical research.

Mayo is the name of a family of doctors, three of whom founded the Mayo Clinic in Rochester, Minn. **William Worrall Mayo** (1819–1911) was born in Manchester, England, and emigrated to the United States. He founded the clinic with his sons **William James** (1861–1939) and **Charles Horace** (1865–1939). The two

sons set up the Mayo Foundation and the Mayo Graduate School of Medicine. Their work was carried on by **Charles William Mayo** (1898–1968), son of Charles Horace.

Minot, George (1885–1950), an American physician, saved the lives of countless patients when he discovered that sufferers from pernicious anemia could be cured if they were given a diet containing large amounts of liver. He served as professor of medicine at Harvard Medical School. Minot and two other doctors, William Murphy and George Whipple, shared the 1934 Nobel prize for medicine for their work on anemia.

Morton, William (1819–1868), a dentist from Boston, Mass., made the first public demonstration of the use of ether as an anesthetic in 1846. He had already used it for extracting a tooth. This demonstration convinced the medical world of the value of anesthesia. He became involved in lawsuit claims about the first use of ether, which ruined him.

Nightingale, Florence (1820–1910), a British nurse, founded the modern nursing profession. Against her parents' wishes, she trained as a nurse and became superintendent of a women's hospital. When the Crimean War began in 1854, she led a band of nurses to the battlefront where wounded soldiers were treated. She revolutionized their care, reducing the death rate from 42 percent to 2 percent. Back in England, she became a semi-invalid, but wrote long reports and persuaded the British government to upgrade its army medical services. Florence Nightingale became a world authority on nursing.

Paracelsus (1493–1541) was the assumed name of a Swiss physician and alchemist, Theophrastus Bombastus von Hohenheim. He introduced a number of drugs into

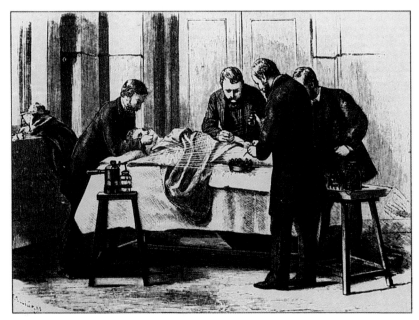

Western medicine, including arsenic, copper sulfate, iron, lead, mercury, opium, and sulfur. Because of his unorthodox methods he was forced to leave Basle.

Paré, Ambroise (c. 1517–1590), was the pioneer of modern surgery. He was in turn a French army surgeon and surgeon to four kings of France. He began the practice of tying off amputation wounds with ligatures instead of cauterizing them with boiling oil. He also recommended massage as a treatment and designed several prostheses (artificial limbs).

Reed, Walter (1851–1902), a U.S. Army doctor, led a medical team to Cuba in 1900 to investigate an outbreak of yellow fever in American forces there. The team proved that the infection was carried by certain mosquitoes, but two of its members died from the fever after being bitten by the insects. The work of Reed's team led to the control of yellow fever in Cuba and Panama.

Roentgen, Wilhelm (1845–1923), a German physicist, won the first Nobel prize in physics for discovering X rays. He was in turn professor of physics at Strasbourg, Giessen, Würzburg, Berlin, and Munich.

Ross, Ronald (1857–1932), a British doctor, discovered that malaria was carried by the anopheles mosquito.

Sabin, Albert (1906–1993), was born in Poland but settled in the United States, where he studied medicine. He introduced the oral vaccine for poliomyelitis in 1960.

Salk, Jonas (1914–1995), an American physician, developed the first vaccine against poliomyelitis in 1953. It had to be given by injection, but its use helped to virtually eliminate polio in many countries. After he discovered the vaccine, Salk devoted the rest of his life to polio research.

Schweitzer, Albert (1875–1965), was a man of many talents, best remembered for his work until 1960 as a medical missionary in Gabon, a French colony in Africa. Schweitzer was born in Alsace, then part of France. He became a brilliant organist, an authority on the works and life of Johann Sebastian Bach, and a preacher. At the age of 30, he began to study medicine and went to Lambaréné in Gabon in 1913. He spent virtually the rest of his life there, tending the sick.

Spock, Benjamin (1903–1998), an American doctor, helped millions of mothers all over the world with his commonsense books about caring for babies and young children, notably *Baby and Child Care* (1946).

Vesalius, Andreas (1514–1564), a Belgian physician, is known as the father of anatomy because of his book on the subject, entitled *On the Fabric of the Human Body*. He graduated from the University of Padua, Italy, where he also taught. He was physician to the Holy Roman Emperor Charles V and his son, Philip II.

Virchow, Rudolf (1821–1902), a German physician, was one of the world's greatest pathologists. He was professor of pathology at Würzburg and Berlin, and then entered politics. He was responsible for improvements in health in Berlin.

Williams, Daniel (1856–1931), founded the Provident Hospital, Chicago, in 1891 so that his fellow blacks could train as doctors and nurses. He was a pioneer of heart surgery and became the first surgeon to mend a heart wound and the membrane around it.

Wright, Louis (1891–1952), triumphed over prejudice against blacks to become director of surgery and president of the medical board at the white Harlem Hospital in New York City. He graduated with honors from Harvard Medical School in 1915. His specialties included head injuries and the use of chemotherapy in treating cancer.

In the early days of X-ray treatment, the dangerous side effects of Roentgen's invention were unknown.

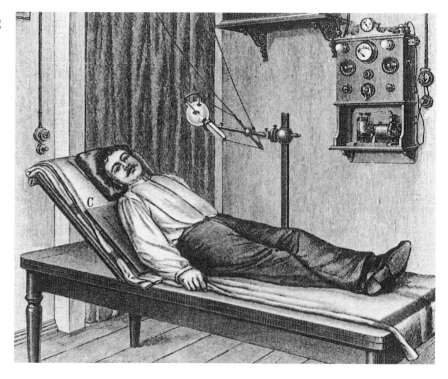

Glossary of Medical Terms

A

ABRASION Superficial grazing of the skin.

ACUTE Any medical condition that has a sudden onset and lasts only a short period of time.

ADHESION Abnormal fibrous connection that forms between abdominal organs, such as the intestines, as a result of inflammation or surgery.

ADIPOSE Relating to animal fat. In humans, the term is applied to connective tissue containing fat. The cells are distended by droplets of fat.

ADRENALIN The body's "fight or flight" hormone, which stimulates the heart, lungs, and other body tissues for action.

AGORAPHOBIA From Greek words meaning "fear of the marketplace;" anxiety which makes people too scared to leave their homes. ▶

ALBINISM An inherited condition leading to a total lack of pigment in the hair, eyes, or skin.

AMINO ACIDS Small chemical molecules containing nitrogen. These are the building blocks that make up all proteins.

ANTACID A medicine, such as bicarbonate of soda, that counteracts the effects of stomach acid and provides relief from indigestion.

AORTIC VALVE The heart valve between the left ventricle (main pumping chamber) and the aorta, the body's major artery.

APOPLEXY An old-fashioned word for a sudden collapse, particularly following a stroke.

APPENDECTOMY An operation to remove an inflamed appendix.

ASPHYXIA The result of oxygen starvation, caused by events such as strangling, smothering, or inhalation of toxic fumes.

ASPIRIN Acetylsalicylic acid; a widely used mild painkiller and anti-inflammatory drug.

ATOPY An allergy characterized by symptoms of asthma, hay fever, and dermatitis.

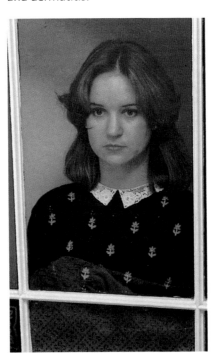

ATRIUM The left atrium and right atrium are the low-pressure pumping chambers of the heart.

ATROPHY Wasting or withering of an organ or tissue.

B

BARIUM A substance that shows up as opaque on an X ray, used to observe the digestive tract.

BCG (Bacillus Calmette-Guerin) A form of bacterium that is able to stimulate immunity without causing disease. It is used in some countries as a vaccination against TB.

BENIGN A term used to describe a condition, usually a tumor, that is relatively harmless and will not spread throughout the body.

BILE Fluid produced by the liver and stored in the gall bladder. Bile enters the intestines through the bile duct.

BIOFEEDBACK A technique in which electronic measurements of bodily functions, such as blood pressure, are used to try to train the body to control the function.

BIOPSY A small tissue sample taken from the body for microscopic examination to determine the nature of the disease process.

BIORHYTHMS Internal body clocks that control physical, emotional, and intellectual cycles.

BLOOD CLOTTING The solidifying of the blood after any damage to stop bleeding.

BLOOD TYPE Blood from another individual is foreign to the body's immune system. Blood typing allows compatible blood to be used for transfusion.

BLUE BABY A baby born with a heart defect that results in a lack of oxygen in the blood.

BOOSTER SHOT Following initial vaccination, booster shots may be given after a few months or years to maintain immunity.

BOWEL Another word for intestine.

BRADYCARDIA A slow heart beat.

C

CAPILLARY The tiny thin-walled blood vessels that connect the arterioles (the ends of the arteries) to the venules (the ends of the veins) and allow the contents of the blood to be passed through to the tissues.

CARBUNCLE A large form of boil with numerous pockets of pus.

CARCINOGEN Substance that can cause cancer.

CARCINOMA The most common form of cancer that occurs in certain cells; in skin, mucous membranes lining organs, and some glands.

CARDIAC ARREST A collapse in which the heart stops beating. The many causes include heart attacks, electrocution, drug overdoses, and drowning.

CATARRH The excessive flow of mucus caused by inflammation of a mucous membrane.

CATHETER A thin tube passed into the body. Bladder catheters, for example, are used to drain urine.

CAUTERIZE The use of heat or strong chemicals to burn areas of bleeding or oozing tissue in order to stop further bleeding.

CELIAC DISEASE A condition leading to poor absorption of food through the intestines; it is caused by sensitivity of the intestine's lining to gluten, found in certain foods, such as wheat flour. It is controlled by removing all gluten from the diet.

CEREBELLUM Part of the brain concerned with coordinating movement and maintaining equilibrium. It lies at the back of the skull, underneath the cerebrum.

CEREBRAL HEMORRHAGE Bleeding into the brain, giving rise to a stroke.

CEREBROSPINAL FLUID Fluid that bathes and cushions the brain and spinal cord.

CERVICAL COLLAR A collar to support the neck after injury or strain.

CHEMOTHERAPY The use of chemical compounds in the treatment of disease, most often used in the treatment of cancers.

CHILBLAINS Hot, red, itchy patches of skin on the toes or fingers caused by exposure to cold.

CHIROPRACTIC A method of treatment based on manipulation of the spine to restore normal nerve function. This is claimed to cure a range of conditions.

CHOLESTEROL A fatty substance that is an essential part of the structure of cell walls. When present in the blood in excessive quantities, it can narrow or block arteries, causing heart attacks, strokes, limb gangrene, and other diseases.

CHROMOSOME ABNORMALITY A condition present from birth that is caused by an abnormal number of chromosomes, or abnormality in the structure of one of them. ▶

CHRONIC Any illness or condition that continues for a long period.

COAGULATION The process in which blood solidifies to form a clot.

CODEINE A painkilling drug of the opium group.

COLIC Pain in the abdomen that comes in waves, building up to a peak, then fading away.

CONGENITAL DISEASE Any disease present from birth.

CONNECTIVE TISSUE The basic cement and packaging of the body, which holds the organs in place and fills spaces. It consists of loose or dense bundles of collagen fibers and many cells in a liquid, gelatinous, or solid medium.

CONTRACEPTION Methods of preventing pregnancy.

CONVALESCENCE The recovery period following an illness or operation during which the patient regains fitness, strength, and energy.

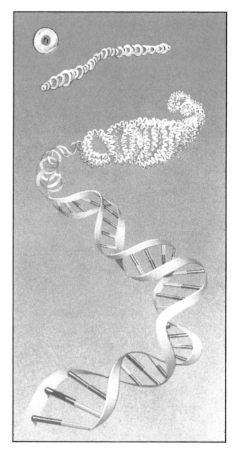

CONVULSION A fit or seizure.

CORNEA The transparent front window of the eye. ▼

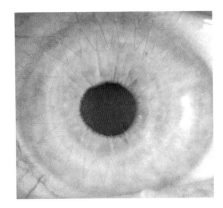

CORPUSCLE An old-fashioned word for a red or a white blood cell.

CORTISONE A hormone produced by the adrenal gland with anti-allergic and anti-inflammatory activity.

CROUP A barking cough and difficulty in breathing, affecting children and caused by nose and throat infection.

CT SCAN (Computerized axial tomography) An X-ray–based technique that builds up detailed pictures of internal structures, producing images representing slices through the body.

CYTOLOGY Study of the body's cells.

CYTOTOXIC DRUGS Drugs that kill cells; used to treat cancers.

D

DECONGESTANT A drug used to reduce congestion (stuffiness) of the air passages.

DEFIBRILLATOR A machine that delivers a sudden, pulsed electric shock to the chest to make the heart resume rhythmical beating.

DEHYDRATION Lack of fluid.

DERMATOLOGIST A doctor who specializes in diseases of the skin.

DETACHED RETINA A condition in which the retina, the light-sensitive layer at the back of the eye, is displaced by fluid collecting behind it.

DIALYSIS A method of taking over the function of the kidneys and keeping the blood free from waste products, usually involving the use of a machine.

DISLOCATION The failure of one part of a joint to meet up with the connecting joint because it has become displaced.

DIURETIC Drugs that increase the loss of water and salt from the kidneys.

DIVERTICULITIS Inflammation of the pouches that form in the colonic wall.

DOWN SYNDROME A condition caused by chromosome abnormality; sufferers are born mentally retarded and they have a distinctive facial appearance.

DROPSY An old-fashioned word for swelling (edema) caused by heart or kidney failure.

DUODENAL ULCER A breakdown in the surface lining of the duodenum caused by stomach acid. ▶

DYSPEPSIA Indigestion usually caused by stomach acid.

DYSURIA Pain on passing urine; a symptom of an infection in the bladder or urethra.

E

ECT (Electroconvulsive therapy) An electrical stimulus across the brain, given under anesthetic, to produce a brief convulsion in the brain. It is only used in rare cases to relieve depression.

EDEMA Swelling of tissues due to an increase in the fluid content. Often seen around the ankles.

ELECTRODE A contact that picks up electrical signals from the surface of the body.

EMBOLISM The blocking of a blood vessel by a substance such as a blood clot or an air bubble.

ENCEPHALITIS An infection that causes inflammation of the brain.

ENDOCARDITIS Infection of the inner surface of the heart, such as the lining of the heart wall or a heart valve.

ENDOCRINE SYSTEM The system of hormones that controls many of the body's chemical processes and the glands that produce them.

ENEMA Fluid passed into the rectum to treat constipation or flush out the lower gut.

ENURESIS Passing urine without control, usually during sleep. The condition occurs mainly in children.

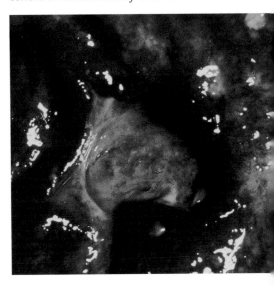

ESOPHAGUS The gullet, which leads from the mouth down through the chest to the stomach.

EUSTACHIAN TUBE The tube that connects the ear to the nasal cavity and throat. It balances the pressure on either side of the eardrum.

EXPECTORANT A medicine that helps you cough up phlegm from the lungs.

F

FISSURE A split in the skin or in any other surface.

FISTULA An abnormal channel between two internal organs, or from an internal organ to the skin.

FIT Uncontrollable twitching or shaking of part or all of the body. It can be caused by epilepsy, fever, head injury, or a brain tumor.

FLAT FOOT Foot that is lacking the normal arch.

FLATULENCE Passing excessive gas by burping or through the rectum.

FONTANELLES The gaps between the developing bones of a baby's skull, covered by soft tissue.

FORENSIC MEDICINE The branch of pathology that deals with unnatural criminal damage or death.

G

GAMMA GLOBULINS Proteins that circulate in the blood and carry antibodies; gamma globulin shots may be given to fight infections.

GANGLION A small cyst that is filled with a jellylike fluid. The ganglion usually occurs on the wrist or the back of the hand. The knots of nerve tissue that act as relay stations in the nervous system are also called ganglions.

GASTRIC ULCER A break in the inner lining of the stomach, caused by excess acidity and a defect in the protective coating of mucus.

GERIATRICS The branch of medical and social science dealing with the health and care of the elderly.

GINGIVITIS Inflammation of the gums, usually due to plaque.

GLUCOSE A simple sugar that is produced by the breakdown of starches and sweet foods. It is the main source of energy for the cells.

GLUTEN A protein found in wheat and wheat products responsible for producing celiac disease.

GLYCOGEN A form of glucose stored in the liver and muscles and released as needed for energy.

GRAFT Transfer of a piece of tissue, such as skin or bone, from another area of the body or from a donor to replace damaged or diseased tissue.

GROWTH A nonmedical term usually referring to a benign or malignant tumor.

H

HALITOSIS Bad or foul-smelling breath.

HAMMER TOE A common deformity, usually affecting the second toe (the one next to the big toe).

HAMSTRING Group of muscles at the back of the thigh.

HEART BLOCK A condition in which the electrical impulses in the heart are blocked. This is usually due to hardening of the coronary arteries, which gives rise to a slow heart rate. Pacemakers are used in treatment.

HEARTBURN A burning sensation behind the breast bone (sternum), caused by stomach acid in the esophagus and relieved by antacids.

HEART COMPRESSION A technique used to support the circulation after the heart has stopped beating and to stimulate the heart back into action. It involves rhythmically pressing downward on the chest at 80–100 times a minute. ▼

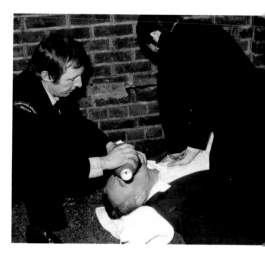

HEART FAILURE Inability of the heart to pump efficiently; as a result, fluid collects in the legs and lungs.

HEAT TREATMENT The application of heat to a diseased or injured area; especially useful for arthritis.

HEMATOMA A collection of blood in the skin, which shows up as a bruise.

HEMATURIA Blood in the urine.

HEMODIALYSIS The use of a kidney machine to remove waste products from the blood after the kidneys have stopped functioning.

HEMOGLOBIN A protein in the red blood cells that carries oxygen from the lungs to all parts of the body.

HYPER- A prefix meaning greater than normal, from the Greek word *hyper*, meaning above.

HYPERBARIC OXYGEN A form of treatment in which oxygen is given at very high pressures. This relieves conditions in which the tissues are lacking oxygen.

HYPO- A prefix usually meaning less than normal, from the Greek word *hypo*, meaning under or below.

HYPOCHONDRIA Neurotic preoccupation with health, with exaggeration of the severity of real or imagined symptoms.

HYPODERMIC Literally, means under (*hypo*) the skin (*dermis*). A hypodermic needle is used to inject drugs under the skin.

HYPOGLYCEMIA An abnormally low level of sugar in the blood. Symptoms include confusion, trembling, and sweating.

HYPOTHALAMUS The area at the base of the brain that controls many of the body's automatic and hormone-related activities.

HYPOTHYROIDISM Underactivity of the thyroid gland leading to weight gain and thick, dry skin.

I

IMPACTED TEETH Teeth that are wedged in position beneath the gum and so fail to grow from the jaw into the mouth properly.

INCONTINENCE Failure to control the activity of either the bowels or the bladder, or both.

INCUBATION PERIOD The period between exposure to a contagious or similar infection and the first appearance of any symptoms.

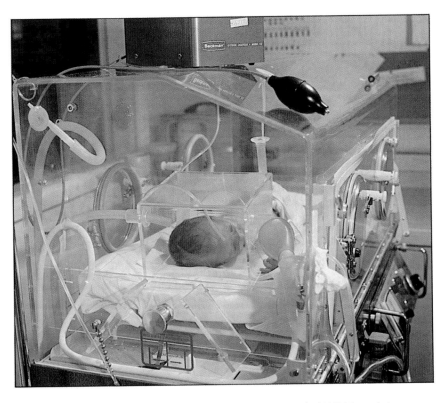

▲ **INCUBATORS** Special protective heated cribs for the care of premature or ill babies after birth.

INFLAMMATION This is a reaction of the tissues of the body to injury or illness, characterized by redness, heat, swelling, and pain; it is a mechanism of defense and repair.

INHALERS Containers that release doses of drugs for inhalation to treat asthma and a variety of other respiratory disorders.

INJECTION Method of delivery of a drug into muscles, veins, or tissues using a hypodermic syringe.

INOCULATION The administration of a vaccine to stimulate production of protective antibodies that results in immunization.

INSOMNIA Difficulties in sleeping.

INTELLIGENCE QUOTIENT (IQ) A numerical scale used to measure a person's intelligence.

INTRAVENOUS (IV) Within or into a vein.

IRRADIATION Exposure to rays such as X rays. Tissue irradiation is used in cancer treatment.

IRRITABLE BOWEL SYNDROME Also known as irritable or spastic colon, this is a condition in which the waves of muscular contraction that move the contents of the intestine are irregular and uncoordinated, leading to nausea, abdominal cramps, and constipation or diarrhea. Stress is a major cause.

J

JUGULAR VEINS Two or more veins draining blood from the head.

K

KELOID An excessive thickening of skin around a scar, caused by a defective healing process.

KERATIN The dead skin cells that make up the outer layers of the skin, the nails, and the hair.

KERATITIS Inflammation of the cornea of the eye.

KETONES Acid waste products from the burning of fats by the body's cells. Ketones are produced in uncontrolled diabetes, since cells have to use fat as fuel when there is insufficient available glucose.

KIDNEY MACHINE A machine that artificially clears the blood of waste products, such as urea, using a process called dialysis.

KNEE JERK A reflex, where the thigh muscles contract sharply to produce a kick. This is a result of the tendon being struck by a light blow with a rubber-covered hammer. ▼

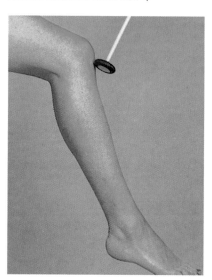

KNOCK-KNEES A minor deformity in which the legs bend inward at the knee so that they appear to knock into each other on walking.

KWASHIORKOR A state of very poor nutrition in children, resulting from a lack of protein.

KYPHOSIS Outward curvature of the spine from front to back. ▶

L

LANCE To cut into an abscess cavity to release the pus.

LAPAROSCOPY The use of a special viewing telescope that is passed through the abdominal or chest wall.

LARYNX The voice box, which contains the vocal cords.

LASERS Sources of pure and critically focusable light that can be used in surgery, especially on eyes.

LESION A general word meaning an abnormality of structure or injury that leads to disruption of function or to disease.

LEUCOCYTOSIS An excess of white cells in the blood, often due to infection.

LEVODOPA A drug that alleviates the effects of Parkinson's disease.

LICHEN PLANUS A skin disease in which the skin thickens and hardens into red patches.

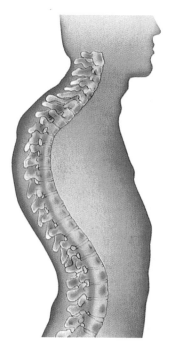

LIGHT TREATMENT Ultraviolet light is used in the treatment of some skin diseases, and blue light in the treatment of jaundiced babies.

LINIMENT A liquid rubbed on the skin to relieve pain in underlying muscles.

LOCAL ANESTHETIC An injection that deadens the nerves and prevents pain in the surrounding area only. ▼

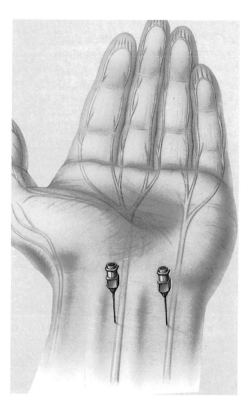

LOIASIS An infestation by loa loa worm, common in West Africa.

LUMBAGO Ache or pain in the lower back, caused by muscular strain.

LUMBAR PUNCTURE The technique of removing cerebrospinal fluid for examination by inserting a needle between two vertebrae and into the canal where the spinal cord lies.

LYMPHOCYTES The main cells of the lymphatic system, which are also found in the blood. They are made in tthe spleen, bone marrow, and thymus and control the body's immune system.

M

MALABSORPTION Failure of the intestine to absorb nutrients.

MALIGNANT Life-threatening.

MALOCCLUSION Failure of the teeth to meet properly on biting.

MANIPULATION A technique that is used to overcome the muscle spasm that gives rise to pain around joints, especially around those in the back.

MARROW The soft matter found in the middle of bones; it plays a vital part in blood formation.

MEMBRANE Any thin sheet of tissue. The cells are surrounded by a wall or membrane, the chemical characteristics of which are central to the way the cells work.

METABOLISM The chemical processes by which the body works.

MORNING SICKNESS Nausea experienced in early pregnancy.

MUCUS The semiliquid substance that coats many of the internal membranes, preventing both damage and infection.

MYCOSIS Infection by fungi.

MYOPATHY Weakness in muscles, not from nerve disease and not inherited. It is due to abnormalities in previously healthy muscle.

N

NATUROPATHY A system of health care that relies on living as naturally as possible and using therapies to help the body cure itself. These include chiropractic, hydrotherapy, massage, and yoga.

NERVES Bundles of specialized conducting tissue that carry messages to and from the brain. Sometimes a disease is said to be due to nerves, when it is thought that it is primarily due to an emotional disturbance rather than a physical one.

NEURALGIA Pain felt along the course of a nerve.

NEUROSURGEON A specialist surgeon who operates on the brain, the spinal cord, and other parts of the nervous system.

NITROUS OXIDE A safe and useful anesthetic gas, sometimes called laughing gas because of its effects.

NUCLEAR MEDICINE The use of radioactive substances to assist in investigation or treatment of disease.

O

OBSTRUCTION A blockage, commonly in the intestines, that leads to distension of the abdomen.

OCCLUSION Literally means a blockage. A thrombosis blocking an artery might be called an occlusion.

ONCOLOGIST A doctor specializing in the treatment of cancer and other related diseases.

OPHTHALMOLOGIST A doctor who specializes in the diagnosis and treatment (sometimes by surgery), of diseases of the eye and associated neurological disorders.

OPHTHALMOSCOPE An instrument that is used to illuminate and inspect the retina at the back of the eye.

OPTIC NERVE Runs from the retina, the light-sensitive membrane of the eye, and carries messages to the brain.

ORTHOPEDICS A branch of surgery concerned with operating on bones and the muscles, tendons, and ligaments that are attached to them. Broken bones (fractures) are treated by orthopedic surgeons.

OSTEOARTHRITIS The wear and tear that leads to distortion and inflammation of some joints.

OSTEOMYELITIS Infection of the bone that destroys tissue. It may be long lasting.

OTITIS Inflammation of the ear. Otitis media, inflammation of the middle ear, is common in children.

P

PACEMAKER An electrical device for dealing with a very slow heartbeat (heart block). A wire is positioned in the heart, and impulses to stimulate the heart muscle are sent down it from a pacing box. ▼

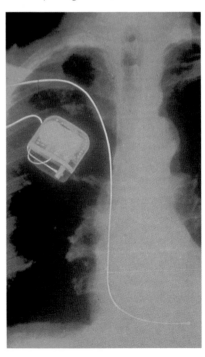

935

PALLIATIVE An operation or form of treatment that is designed to relieve symptoms rather than cure the cause of them.

PALPATE The word doctors use to describe the technique of feeling for abnormalities with their hands during physical examination.

PALPITATION The sensation of the heart beating either very fast or very powerfully, or missing beats. This sensation is sometimes associated with a disorder of the heart's rhythm but is more commonly due to stress or anxiety.

PALSY An old-fashioned word to describe paralysis. Today, it is most often used to describe paralysis of the facial muscles.

PARAPLEGIA Paralysis of the legs as a result of disease or injury in the spinal cord.

PARATHYROID The four parathyroid glands are found behind the thyroid gland. They control calcium levels in the body.

PAROXYSM A term to describe a sudden attack of a symptom, or a spasm or convulsion.

PATHOGEN An infecting organism that causes tissue damage or inflammation.

PEAK FLOW METER An instrument that measures the speed at which air can be blown out, helping to assess the severity of disease in asthma.

PEDIATRICIAN A doctor specializing in the treatment of children.

PEPTIC ULCER The erosion of part of the membrane lining either the stomach or the duodenum. This erosion can be a result of the effects of excess stomach acid.

PERCEPTION The process of receiving information about the outside world by the sensory organs, especially the eyes and ears, and processing it to build up a picture of the world.

PERCUSSION A diagnostic method involving tapping the chest to find out the condition of internal organs.

PERFORATION A hole in an organ caused by disease.

pH The scale of measurement used to assess acidity.

PHALANGES The small bones that are joined together to make the fingers and toes.

PHARYNX The upper part of the throat at the back of the mouth and the nose.

PHLEGM Mucus produced by the nose and sinuses, or by the airways in the chest.

PLACEBO A medicine or tablet that has no effect on the body's processes but has a beneficial effect through the power of suggestion. Placebos are very important in the investigation of drugs, since active substances can be compared with them for efficiency.

PLATELETS The tiny cell fragments that are present in large numbers in the blood. Platelets are essential for normal blood clotting.

PODIATRY Care of the feet, such as the removal of hard skin, corns, and calluses, and care of the toenails.

POLLEN COUNT A count of the number of pollen particles in the air that provides a warning of the risk of symptoms for hay fever sufferers.

POSTMORTEM Literally, after death. An examination of the body after death so that the direct inspection of the organs and the microscopic examination of tissue specimens will help to explain the cause of death or some aspects of the final illness. Postmortem examinations are one of the most important ways in which medical knowledge can be expanded.

PREMEDICATION Drugs that are given to people in order to relax them before surgery.

PROGNOSIS The outlook for a patient; while diagnosis involves the doctor saying what a disease is, prognosis involves saying what the long-term effects will be.

PROLAPSE The failure of an organ to stay in its normal position.

PROPHYLACTIC A measure or form of treatment designed to stop something from happening. For example, a condom may be used to prevent conception or disease.

PROSTAGLANDINS Chemical compounds that act as messengers in the body. Prostaglandins perform a variety of hormonelike actions, such as controlling blood pressure and smooth muscle contraction.

PROSTHESIS Any artificial replacement for a part of the body.

PSYCHOLOGY The study of mind and behavior in relation to a specified field of knowledge or activity.

PYORRHEA Inflammation and infection of the gums.

PYREXIA The medical word for a fever or raised temperature.

Q

Q FEVER This is caused by an organism passed from animals, such as sheep, cattle, and goats, to humans.

QUADRIPLEGIA The paralysis of arms, legs, and the trunk. The condition is caused by severe damage in the neck region.

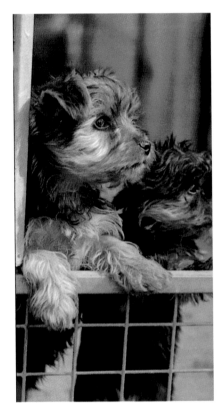

▲ **QUARANTINE** Keeping people or animals isolated because of the risk of catching or passing on an infectious disease.

R

RADIOLOGIST A specialist in the use of X rays or ultrasound, who produces pictures of internal structures and so assists in the diagnosis of disease.

REFERRED PAIN The sensation of pain felt in part of the body that is some distance away from the actual source of the pain.

REFRACTORY A term commonly used by doctors to describe a condition that fails to respond to treatment.

REJECTION OF TISSUE The attacking of foreign tissue by the body's immune system. Rejection is the main risk in transplantation.

RELAPSE The return of an illness after recovery appears to have started.

REMISSION A period free from the symptoms of a chronic illness.

RHESUS (Rh) FACTOR An inherited blood group indicator on the surface of the red blood cells, which is incompatible with blood lacking this factor. A fetus with a different group from that of its mother may have its blood attacked by antibodies.

RHEUMATISM Although not a strict medical term any more, the word *rheumatism* refers to various aches and pains that occur in the body's joints and muscles.

RODENT ULCER A spot or ulcer, usually on the face, which is a mild form of cancer capable of eating away tissue unless it is removed.

ROSEOLA A minor and common viral infection in children and babies, which causes a rash.

RUPTURE Literally, a break. A rupture can occur in the tendons, ligaments, distorted veins, eardrum, and the spleen. Hernias are often referred to as ruptures.

S

SALINE A saltwater solution, commonly used to give fluid intravenously through a drip.

SALIVA The fluid present in the mouth and secreted by the salivary glands.

SANATORIUM A special hospital for the treatment and convalescence of people suffering from chronic disease such as tuberculosis.

SARCOMA A malignant tumor in muscle, bone, or connective tissue. ▼

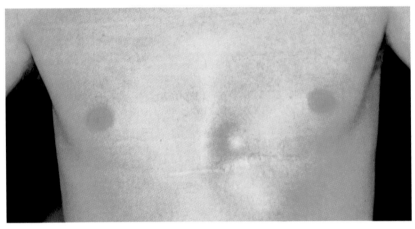

SEBUM The oily substance produced by the sebaceous glands.

SECRETION The production by a gland of a substance (a secretion) that works outside the gland itself.

SENSITIZATION The exposure of the body to a substance, with the result that there is an allergic reaction on subsequent exposures.

SEPTICEMIA A condition where bacteria live and multiply in the blood.

SIDE EFFECT An effect produced by a drug other than the effect for which it is given; for example, drowsiness can be a side effect of antihistamine drugs given for hay fever.

SKIN GRAFT Skin that is transplanted from one part of the body to another to repair damage or to correct a congenital deformity.

SLEEPING SICKNESS The common name for the tropical disease trypanosomiasis, which induces coma.

SOLAR PLEXUS A large, ray-like network of autonomic nerves behind the stomach in the upper abdomen. A lay term used to describe the general area at the top of the abdomen.

SOPORIFIC Something that makes you drowsy or sleepy.

SPASM A strong and involuntary contraction of muscles.

SPASTICITY A neurological term used to describe weakness in a limb due to a problem in the higher parts of the nervous system; the muscles do not relax properly but remain partly contracted.

SPECIMEN Any sample of a tissue, body secretion, or body fluid.

SPECULUM An instrument that can be inserted into a body opening in order to examine it.

SPUTUM The secretions of the bronchial tubes, which increase in volume when infection is present and may be colored by the presence of dead bacteria.

STERILE ENVIRONMENT An area kept as free as possible from bacteria, to reduce the risk of infection.

STERILIZATION The process of making surgical instruments bacteria-free for operations; also an operation to prevent conception.

STEROIDS Complex chemical molecules such as cortisone and drugs that have a similar effect.

STETHOSCOPE Instrument used for listening to the sounds of the heart, lungs, and other internal organs. ▼

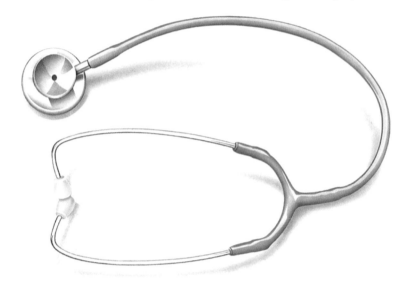

STREPTOCOCCUS A type of bacterium that often causes throat infections.

STREPTOMYCIN An antibiotic used mainly against tuberculosis.

STRICTURE Abnormal narrowing in a tube, especially used to describe constriction in the intestine and in the urinary tract.

SUBCUTANEOUS Under the skin.

SUBLINGUAL Literally, under the tongue. It is one of the routes by which drugs may be given.

SUPPOSITORIES Drugs made in a form to be inserted into the anus.

SUPPURATION The production of pus as a result of infection.

SUTURE The medical name for a stitch used to close a wound or an incision.

SYNCOPE Sudden loss of consciousness. It is also known as fainting.

SYNDROME Literally, running together; the appearance of a number of signs and symptoms occurring together in a discernible pattern that is characteristic of a particular disorder.

SYRINGE A device with a barrel and plunger that is used for many purposes, including giving shots.

T

TENNIS ELBOW Inflammation of tendons on the outer side of the elbow. This may be the result of overuse of the arm. ▼

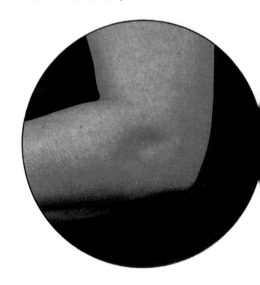

TENOSYNOVITIS Inflammation of the lubricated sheaths through which some tendons run, for example, those running across the wrist. It occurs when a repetitive activity becomes so excessive that the tendon sheath cannot lubricate the tendon within it sufficiently.

THERMOGRAPHY A technique that produces pictures of the body in which different colors represent areas of different temperature.

THROMBOSIS The formation of a blood clot or thrombus, where it occurs abnormally within an artery or a vein due to a damaged lining.

THROMBUS A clot of blood.

TINEA Skin infection with fungus, such as athlete's foot.

TINNITUS Ringing or buzzing sounds in the ears.

TISSUE CULTURE Growing animal or human tissue outside the body.

TISSUE TYPING Tissue, like blood, has various types; tissue typing is essential when transplanting organs to reduce the risk of rejection.

TOLERANCE Accustoming the body to a drug that then has less effect.

TONIC A nonspecific medicine or herbal mixture that aims to produce a general improvement in health and function.

TONSILLECTOMY An operation to remove the tonsils.

TOPICAL APPLICATION The application of a drug straight onto the skin in the form of a lotion, cream, or ointment.

TOXEMIA Bacterial toxins (poisons) in the bloodstream, which can lead to toxic shock syndrome.

TOXICOLOGY The study of the nature and biological effects of poisoning, as well as its treatment.

TRACHEOSTOMY The opening that is made through the neck into the windpipe to aid breathing. Tracheotomy is the name of the surgical procedure that is used to make the opening.

TRACTION The pulling of broken bones into place by a system of ropes, pulleys, and weights.

TRANSFUSION Feeding a substance such as blood into a vein, directly into the bloodstream.

TRAUMA This Greek word meaning damage is used for both emotional shock and physical injury.

TREMOR The involuntary trembling of some part of the body.

U

ULTRASOUND The use of very high frequency sound waves to produce images of internal structures. It works on the same principle as the sonar used to detect submarines. ▼

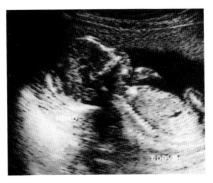

URINALYSIS The testing of urine for abnormal substances such as sugar, blood, or protein.

URINE The fluid produced by the kidneys, containing excess water and waste products built up in the body.

V

VACCINATION The administration of a vaccine, usually via a shot, to prevent an infectious disease.

VALIUM (Diazepam) A very widely used tranquilizer.

VALVE A mechanism that allows fluid to flow only one way through a tube. The most important valves control blood flow in the heart.

VEIN The veins are thin-walled vessels that return blood from the tissues to the heart.

VERRUCA A wart on any part of the skin. A localized, abnormal but benign overgrowth of skin cells that is caused by the human papilloma virus.

VIRULENT A term used to describe a virus or bacterium that produces severe symptoms.

VITAL CAPACITY The total amount of air someone can breathe into the lungs after breathing out to the fullest possible extent.

W

WASTING Loss of muscle tissue as a result of lack of use, especially if the nerve supply to the muscle has failed.

WATER ON THE KNEE Excessive production of fluid in the synovial membrane lining the knee joint.

X

X RAYS These rays are a form of electromagnetic radiation and are used to help with diagnosis. When X rays are passed through the body, the bones show as white, while the soft tissues, such as muscles, appear as shades of gray.

Pronunciation Guide

A

Abdomen, AB duh mun *or*
ab DOH mun
Abortion, uh BAWR shun
Abrasions, uh BRAY zhunz
Abscess, AB ses
Acne, AK nee
Acupuncture, AK yuh punk chur
Addiction, uh DIK shun
Adenoids, AD uh noydz
Adolescence, AD uh LES uns
Adoption, uh DOP shun
Adrenal glands, uh DREE nul
GLANDZ
Aerobics, e ROH bix
Aerosols, ER uh sawlz
Aging, AY jing
AIDS, AYDZ
Alcohol, AL kuh hawl
Alcoholism, AL kuh hawl ih zum
Alimentary canal, al uh MEN tur ee
kuh NAL
Allergies, AL ur jeez
Alternative medicine,
awl TUR nuh tiv MED uh sin
Alzheimer's disease, AWLT zye murz
di ZEEZ
Amebic dysentery, uh MEE bik
DIS un ter ee
Amnesia, am NEE zee uh
Amphetamines, am FET uh meenz
Amputation, am pyoo TAY shun
Analgesics, an ul JEE zix
Anatomy, uh NAT uh mee
Anemia, uh NEE mee uh
Anesthesiologist,
an us THEE zee AHL uh jist
Anesthetics, an us THET ix
Aneurysm, AN yuh riz um
Angina, an JEYE nuh
Animals, AN uh mulz
Anorexia nervosa, an uh REK see uh
nur VOH suh
Antacids, ant AS idz
Anthrax, AN thraks
Antibiotics, an ti bye AHT ix
Antibody and antigen, AN ti bahd ee
and AN tuh jin
Antihistamine, an ti HIS tuh meen
Antiseptics, an ti SEP tix

Anxiety, ang ZYE uh tee
Aphasia, uh FAY zee uh
Appendicitis, uh PEN duh SYE tus
Appetite, AP uh tyte
Artery, AHR tur ee
Artery diseases and disorders,
AHR tur ee di ZEE zuz and
dis AWR durz
Arthritis, ahr THRYT is
Artificial, ahr tuh FISH ul
Asbestosis, az bes TOH sis
Aspirin, AS pur in
Asthma, AZ muh
Astigmatism, uh STIG muh tiz um
Atherosclerosis,
ath ur oh skluh ROH sis
Athlete's foot, ATH leets fuht
Atrium, AY tree um
Autism, AW tiz um

B

Bacillary dysentery, BAS il er ee
DIS en ter ee
Backache, BAK ayk
Backbone, BAK bon
Bacteremia, bak tir EE mee uh
Bacteria, bak TEER ee uh
Bacterial diseases, bak TIR ee uhl
di ZEE zuz
Bad breath, BAD BRETH
Balance, BA luns
Baldness, BAWLD nes
Barbiturates, bahr BICH ur its
Basal metabolism, BAY sul
muh TAB uh liz um
Bedbugs, BED bugz
Bedsores, BED sohrz
Bedwetting, BED weh ting
Bee stings, BEE stingz
Behavior, bi HAYV yur
Behavior therapy, bi HAYV yur
THER uh pee
Beriberi, ber ee BER ee
Bile, BYEL
Bilharzia, bil hahr ZEYE uh
Biorhythms, BYE oh ridh umz
Birth, burth
Birth control, BURTH kun TROHL
Birth defects, BURTH dee FEKTS
Birthmarks, BURTH marx

Bites and stings, BYTES and STINGZ
Blackheads, BLAK hedz
Bladder, BLAD ur
Blastomycosis,
BLAS toh mye KOH sis
Blindness, BLYND nes
Blisters, BLIS turz
Blood, BLUHD
Blood poisoning, BLUHD
POY zun ing
Blood pressure, BLUHD
PRESH ur
Blood transfusion, BLUHD
trans FYOO zhun
Blood type, BLUHD TYEP
Blushing, BLUSH ing
Body odor, BAHD ee OH dur
Boils, BOY uhlz
Bone, BOHN
Botulism, BAHCH uh liz um
Bowel, BOW ul
Brain, BRAYN
Breast, BREST
Breathing, BREE THING
Bronchitis, brahng KYTE is
Brucellosis, brooh sul OH sis
Bruises, BROOHZ ez
Bubonic plague, byoo BAHN ik
PLAYG
Bulimia, boo LEEM ee uh
Bunions, BUN yunz
Bursitis, bur SYTE is

C

Caffeine, kaf EEN
Calcium, KAL see um
Calories, KAL ur eez
Cancer, KAN sur
Candida, KAN dih duh
Cannabis, KAN uh bis
Capillary, KAP il er ee
Carbohydrates,
kahr buh HYE drayts
Carbon monoxide poisoning,
KAHR bun mahn OK syde
POY zuh ning
Cartilage, KART ul ij
Cataract, KAT uh rakt
Cells and chromosomes, selz and
KROH muh sohmz

Cerebral palsy, SER uh bruhl (*or*
suh REE brul) PAWL zee
Cervix, SUR vix
Cesarean section, seh ZAR ee un
SEK shun
Chagas disease, SHA gus di zeez
Chemotherapy,
kee moh THER uh pee
Chiggers, CHIG erz
Chilblains, CHIL blaynz
Chiropractic, KYE roh prak tik
Chlamydia, kluh MID ee ah
Choking, CHO king
Cholera, KAHL ur uh
Cholesterol, kuh LES tuh rohl
Circulatory system,
SUR kyuh luh tor ee SIS tum
Cirrhosis, suh ROH sis
Cleft palate, KLEFT PAL it
Cocaine, koh KAYN
Colon, KOH lun
Coma, KOH muh
Communicable diseases,
kuh MYOOH nuh kuh bul
di ZEE zuz
Condom, KAHN dum
Conjunctivitis,
kun jungk tuh VYTE is
Constipation, kahn stuh PAY shun
Contagious diseases, kun TAY jus
di ZEE zuz
Contraception, kahn trah SEP shun
Coronary thrombosis,
KAWR uh ner ee thrahm BOH sis
Cosmetics, kahz MET ix
Coughing, CAW fing
Cramps, KRAMPS
Cretinism, KRE tin ih zum
Cults, KUHLTS
Cuticle, KYEW tih kul
Cuts and abrasions, KUHTS and
uh BRAY zhunz
Cysts, SISTS
Cystic fibrosis, SIS tik fye BROH sis
Cystitis, sis TYT is

D

Dandruff, DAN druff
Deafness, DEF nes
Death, DETH
Delirium, di LIR ee um
Dementia, di MEN shuh
Dengue fever, DEN gay FEE vur
Dental care, DEN tul KAR
Dentist, DEN tist

Deodorants and antiperspirants,
dee OH dur unts and
an tee PUR spir ents
Deoxyribonucleic acid,
dee OX ee REYE boh noo KLEE ik
AS id
Depression, di PRESH un
Dermatitis, dur muh TYTE is
Detoxification, dee tahks if ih KAY
shun
Diabetes, dye uh BEET is *or*
dye uh BEET eez
Diagnosis, dye ug NOH sis
Diaphragm, DYE uh fram
Diarrhea, dye uh REE uh
Diet, DYE ut
Digestive system, di JES tiv SIS tum
Diphtheria, dip THIR ee uh
Disinfectants and antiseptics,
dis in FEK tunts and an ti SEP tix
Dislocation, dis loh KAY shun
Dizziness, DI zee nes
Dog bites, DAWG BEYTS
Down syndrome, DOWN
SIN drohm
Dreaming, DREE ming
Duodenal ulcer, doo uh DEE nul UL
sur
Dyslexia, dis LEK see uh

E

Ear and hearing, EER and HEE ring
Earwax, EER waks
Eczema, EK suh muh *or* ig ZEE muh
Elbow, EL boh
Electric shock, i LEK trik SHAHK
Electrocardiogram,
i lek troh KAHR dee uh gram
Electroencephalogram,
i lek troh en SEF uh luh gram
Emergency medical identification,
i MUR jun see MED i kul
eye den tu fih KAY shun
Emotions, i MOH shunz
Emphysema, em fuh SEE muh
Encephalitis, en sef uh LYTE is
Endocarditis, en doh kahr DYE tis
Endocrine system, EN duh krin
SIS tum
Environment, in VYE run munt
Environmental diseases,
in VYE run MEN tul di ZEE zuz
Enzymes, EN zymz
Epidemic, ep uh DEM ik
Epilepsy, EP uh lep see

Esophagus, i SAHF uh gus
Estrogen, ES truh jun
Ethical issues, ETH i kul ISH ooz
Euthanasia, yooh thuh NAY see uh
Exercise, EK sur syze
Exocrine glands, EX uh krin
GLANDZ
Exposure, ik SPOH zhur

F

Face, FAYS
Fainting, FAYN ting
Faith healing, FAYTH hee ling
Falls, FAWLZ
Family life, FAM uh lee LEYF
Family therapy, FAM uh lee
THER uh pee
Fatigue, fuh TEEG
Fear, FEER
Feminine hygiene, FEM uh nin
HYE jeen
Fertility, fur TIL uh tee
Fever, FEE vur
Fibrillation, fib ruh LAY shun
Fibroids, FEYE broydz
Fibromyalgia,
FEYE broh my Al jee uh
Filariasis, FiL ahr EYE uh sis
Flatulence, FLACH oo luns
Fleas, FLEEZ
Flu, FLOOH
Flukes, FLOOKS
Fluoridation, flu awr uh DAY shun
Food and nutrition, FOOD and
noo TRISH un
Food additives, FOOD AD uh tivz
Food poisoning, FOOD
POY zun ing
Fracture and dislocation,
FRAK chur and dis loh KAY shun
Frostbite, FRAWST byt
Fungal infections, FUNG gul
in FEK shunz

G

Gall bladder, GAWL bla dur
Gallstones, GAWL stohnz
Gangrene, GANG green
Gastric ulcer, GAS trik UL sur
Gastritis, gas TRYTE is
Genes, jeenz
Genetics, juh NET iks
German measles, JUR mun
MEE zulz
Gigantism, JEYE gan ti zum

Gingivitis, jin juh VYTE is
Glandular fever, GLAND juh lur
FEE vur
Glaucoma, glaw KOH muh
Goiter, GOYT ur
Gonorrhea, gahn uh REE uh
Gout, GOWT
Grief, GREEF
Group therapy, GROOP
THER uh pee
Gynecologist, gye nuh KAHL uh jist

H

Halitosis, hal uh TOH sis
Hallucinations,
huh LOOH suh nay shunz
Hallucinogens,
huh LOOH suh nuh jenz
Handicaps, HAN dee kaps
Hansen's disease, HAN sunz
di ZEEZ
Hay fever, HAY FEE vur
Headache, HED ayk
Healing, HEE ling
Heimlich maneuver, HYME lik
muh NOOH vur
Hemophilia, hee muh FIL ee uh
Hemorrhage, HEM uh rij
Hemorrhoids, HEM uh roydz
Hepatitis, hep uh TYTE is
Herbal remedies, HUR bul (or
Ur bul) REM uh deez
Heredity, huh RED uh tee
Hernia, HUR nee uh
Heroin, HER uh win
Herpes, HUR peez
Hiccups, HIK ups
Histoplasmosis,
HIS toh plaz MOH sis
Hives, HYVES
Hodgkin's disease, HOJ kinz
di ZEEZ
Hookworm disease, HOOK wurm
di ZEEZ
Hormones, HAWR mohnz
Hormonal disorders, hor MOH nul
dis AWR durz
Hospice, HAHS pis
Hydatid disease, HYE duh tid
di ZEEZ
Hydrocephalus,
HYE druh SEF uh lus
Hygiene, HYE jeen
Hyperactivity, HYE pur ak TIV it ee
Hypertension, HYE pur TEN shun

Hyperventilation,
HYE pur ven tul LAY shun
Hypnosis, hip NOH sis
Hypnotic drugs, hip NAHT ik
DRUGZ
Hypochondria,
HYE puh KON dree uh
Hypoglycemia,
HYE po gly SEE mee uh
Hypothermia,
HYE puh THIR mee uh
Hysteria, his TER ee uh

I

Immune system, i MYOOHN
SIS tum
Immunodeficiency,
i MYOOHN oh di FISH un see
Immunization,
i myoohn eye ZAY shun
Immunosuppressive drugs,
i MYOOHN oh suh PRES iv
DRUGZ
Impetigo, im puh TYE goh
Indigestion, in di JES chun
Indoctrination,
in dahk truh NAY shun
Infectious diseases, in FEK shus
di ZEE zus
Infectious mononucleosis,
in FEK shus
MAHN oh noo klee OH sis
Influenza, in floo EN zuh
Injection, in JEK shun
Insanity, in SAN uh tee
Insects, IN sekts
Insecticides, in SEK tuh sydz
Insomnia, in SAHM nee uh
Insulin, IN suh lin
Intelligence, in TEL uh jens
Intensive care unit, in TEN siv KAYR
YOOH nit
Interferon, in tur FIR ahn
Intestines, in TES tinz
Intoxication,
in TAHK suh KAY shun
Intrauterine device,
in truh YOOH ter in di VYSE
Intravenous therapy,
in truh VEE nus THER uh pee
Iodine, EYE uh dyne
Isometric exercises,
eye suh MET rik EK sur sye
zuz
Itches, ICH uz

J

Jaundice, JAWN dis
Joint, JOYNT
Joint diseases and disorders,
JOYNT di ZEE zuz and
dis AWR durz
Junk food, JUNGK FOOD

K

Kidney, KID nee
Kidney diseases and disorders,
KID nee di ZEE zuz and
dis AWR durz
Knee, NEE
Kyphosis, key FOH sis

L

Larynx, LAR ingks
Lassa fever, LAH suh FEE vur
Laxatives, LAK suh tivz
Lead poisoning, LED POY zuh ning
Learning, LUR ning
Legionnaires' disease,
lee juh NERZ di ZEEZ
Leisure, LEE zhur
Leprosy, LEP ruh see
Leptospirosis, LEP toh spir OH sis
Leukemia, looh KEE mee uh
Leukocytosis,
LOOH koh sye TOH sis
Leukorrhea, looh kor EE uh
Lice, LEYS
Lichen, LEYE kun
Ligaments, LIG uh munts
Liver, LIV ur
Lordosis, lohr DOH sis
Lou Gehrig's disease, LOO
GAYR igz di ZEEZ
Louse, LOWS
Lupus erythematosus, LOO pus
ur ih thi muh TOH sus
Lyme disease, LYME di ZEEZ
Lymphatic system, lim FAT ik
SIS tum
Lysergic acid, lye SUR jik AS id

M

Macrobiotic diet,
ma croh bye AHT ic DYE ut
Malaria, muh LAYR ee uh
Malignancy, muh LIG nun see
Malnutrition, mal noo TRI shun
Manic depression, MAN ik di
PRESH un
Marijuana, mar uh WAH nuh

Marrow, MAR oh
Massage. muh SAHZH
Mastoiditis, mas toy DYE tis
Masturbation, mas tur BAY shun
Measles, MEE zulz
Medicines, MED uh sinz
Melanin, MEL uh nin
Melanoma, mel uh NOH muh
Memory, MEM ur ee
Meningitis, men in JYTE is
Menopause, MEN uh pawz
Menstrual disorders, MEN stru ul dis
AWR durz
Menstruation, men stru AY shun
Mental health, MEN tul HELTH
Mental illness, MEN tul IL nes
Mental retardation, MEN tul ree tahr
DAY shun
Mercury poisoning, MUR kyoor ee
POY zuh ning
Mescaline, MES kuh leen
Metabolic disorders,
met uh BAHL ik dis AWR durz
Metabolism, muh TAB uh liz um
Metal poisoning, MET ul POY zuh
ning
Methadone, METH uh dohn
Microsurgery,
MYE kroh SUR juh ree
Migraine, MYE grayn
Minerals, MIN ur ulz
Miscarriage, MIS kar ij
Mite, MYTE
Mononucleosis,
MAHN no nooh klee OH sis
Monosodium glutamate,
mahn no SOH dee um
GLOO tuh mayt
Morphine, MAWR feen
Mosquito bites, mus KEET oh
byts
Motion sickness, MOH shun
SIK nus
Mouth, MOWTH
Mouth to mouth resuscitation,
MOWTH to MOWTH
ri sus uh TAY shun
Mucus, MYOOH kus
Multiple sclerosis, MUL tuh pul
skluh ROH sis
Muscles, MUS ulz
Muscular dystrophy, MUS kyuh lur
DIS truh fee
Mutation, myooh TAY shun
Mutism, MYOOH tiz um

Myasthenia gravis,
mye us THEE nee uh GRAH vis
Myocardial infarction, MYE oh KAHR
di ul in FAHRK shun
Myopia, mye OH pee uh

N

Nails, NAYLZ
Narcotics, nar KAHT iks
Nasal congestion, NAY sul
kun JES chun
Nausea, NAW zee uh *or* NAW zhuh
Nephritis, ne FRYTE is
Nervous system, NUR vus SIS tum
Neuritis, noo RYTE us
Neurologist, noo RAHL uh jist
Neurosis, no ROH sis
Nicotine, NIK uh teen
Noise, NOYZ
Nonspecific urethritis,
nahn spi SIF ik yoo ree THRYT is
Nose, NOHZ
Nosebleed, NOHZ bleed
Numbness, NUM nus
Nurses, NUR suz
Nursing home, NUR sing HOHM
Nutrition, noo TRISH un
Nutritional disorders,
noo TRISH un ul dis AWR durz

O

Obesity, oh BEE si tee
Obsessive-compulsive neurosis,
ub SES iv-kum PUL siv noo ROH sis
Obstetrician, ahb stuh TRISH un
Occupational hazards,
ahk yuh PAY shun ul HAZ urdz
Ophthalmologist, ahf thul MAHL uh
jist
Opium and opiates, OH pee um
and OH pee uts
Organ, AWR guhn
Orthodontics, awr thuh DAHN
tiks
Osteoarthritis,
AHS tee oh ahr THRYTE is
Osteosarcoma,
AHS tee oh sahr KOH muh
Osteopath, AHS tee uh path
Osteoporosis, AHS tee oh por OH
sis
Otitis, oh TYTE us
Ovaries and ovulation, OH vur eez
and ahv yuh LAY shun
Oxygen, AHK si jun

P

Paget's disease, PAJ ets di ZEEZ
Pain, PAYN
Palate, PAL it
Pancreas, PAN kree us
Panic, PAN ik
Pap smear, PAP smeer
Paralysis, pu RAL uh sis
Paranoid disorders, PAR uh noyd
dis AWR durz
Paraplegia, par uh PLEE jee uh
Parasites and parasitic diseases,
PAR uh sytes and par uh SIH tik
di ZEEZ us
Parathyroid gland,
par uh THYE royd GLAND
Parkinson's disease,
PAHR kin sunz di ZEEZ
Pathologist, puh THAHL uh jist
Pediatrician, pee dee uh TRISH un
Pellagra, puh LAG ruh
(*or* puh LAY grah)
Pelvis, PEL vus
Penicillin, pen uh SIL un
Penis, PEE nis
Peptic ulcer, PEP tik UL sur
Peripheral nervous system,
puh RIH fer ul NUR vus SIS tum
Peritonitis, per i tuh NYTE is
Pernicious anemia, pur NISH us
uh NEE mee uh
Peroxide, pur AHK syde
**Personality and personality
disorders**, pur suh NAL uh tee
and pur suh NAL uh tee
dis AWR durs
Pesticides, PES tuh sydez
Pharmacist, FAHR muh sist
Pharmacologist,
fahr muh KAHL uh jist
Pharynx, FAR ingks
Phlebitis, fli BYTE is
Phobias, FOH bee ahz
Physical examination, FIZ i kul
ig zam uh NAY shun
Physical fitness, FIZ i kul FIT nus
Physical therapy, FIZ i kul
THER uh pee
Physician, fiz I shun
Pigeon toes, PIH jun tohz
Pigmentation, pig men TAY shun
Pinworms, PIN wurmz
Pituitary gland, pit TOOH uh ter ee
GLAND
Placebo, pluh SEE boh

Plague, PLAYG
Plaque, PLAK
Plasma, PLAZ muh
Plastic surgery, PLAS tik SUR jur ee
Pleurisy, PLOOR uh see
Pneumoconiosis, noo moh kon ee OH sis
Pneumonia, noo MOHN yuh
Podiatrist, puh DYE uh trist
Poison and poisoning, POY zun and POY zuh ning
Poisonous plants, POY zuh nous PLANTS
Poliomyelitis, POH lee oh mye uh LYTE us
Pollution, puh LOO shun
Polyp, PAHL ip
Posture, PAHS chur
Potassium, Puh TAS ee um
Pregnancy, PREG nun see
Premature birth, pree muh TOOR BURTH
Premenstrual syndrome, pree MEN strul SIN drohm
Preventive medicine, Pri VEN tiv MED uh sin
Progesterone, pro JEST ur ohn
Prostate gland, PRAHS tayt GLAND
Prosthesis, prahs THEE sis
Protein, PROH teen
Psittacosis, sit uh KOH sis
Psoriasis, suh RYE uh sis
Psychiatrist, suh KYE uh trist
Psychoanalysis, SYE koh uh NAL uh sis
Psychosis, sye KOH sis
Psychosomatic disorders, SYE koh soh MAT ik dis AWR durz
Psychotherapist, SYE koh THER uh pist
Puberty, PYOOH bur tee
Public health, PUB lik HELTH
Pulmonary disease, PUL muh ner ee or POOL muh ner ee di ZEEZ
Pulse, PULS
Pyorrhea, pye uh REE uh

Q

Quackery, KWAK uh ree
Quadriplegia, KWAWD ruh PLEE jee uh
Quarantine, KWAWR un teen

R

Rabies, RAY beez
Radiation sickness, ray dee AY shun SIK nus
Radiation therapy, ray dee AY shun THER uh pee
Rape, RAYP
Raynaud's disease, ray NOHZ di ZEEZ
Recreation, rek ree AY shun
Reflexes, REE flek ses
Rehabilitation, ree huh bil uh TAY shun
Rejection, ri JEK shun
Relationships, ri LAY shun ships
Relaxation, ree lak SAYE shun
Reproduction, ree pruh DUK shun
Reproductive system, female, ree pruh DUK tuv SIS tum, FEE mayl
Reproductive system, male, ree pruh DUK tuv SIS tum, MAYL
Rescue breathing, RES kyooh BREE THING
Respiratory system, RES pur uh tawr ee SIS tum
Resuscitation, ri sus uh TAY shun
Reye's syndrome, RAYZ SIN drohm
Rhesus factor, REE sus FAK tur
Rheumatic fever, roo MAT ik FEE vur
Rheumatoid arthritis, ROOH muh toyd ahr THRYTE is
Rhinitis, rye NYTE is
Rib cage, RIB KAYJ
Rickets, RI kets
Rickettsial diseases, ri KET see uhl di ZEEZ uz
Ringworm, RING wurm
Roundworm, ROWND wurm
Rubella, rooh BEL uh

S

Salmonella, sal muh NEL uh
Scabies, SKAY beez
Scarlet fever, SKAHR lit FEE vur
Schistosomiasis, SHIS toh suh MEY uh sis
Schizophrenia, Skit suh FREEN ee uh (or skit suh FREN nee uh)
Sciatica, sye AT i kuh
Scoliosis, skoh lee OH sis
Scurvy, SKUR vee
Sebaceous glands, si BAY shus GLANDZ

Sedatives, SED uh tivz
Senses, SEN sus
Separation, sep uh RAY shun
Sex, SEKS
Sexuality, sex yoo ALL uh tee
Sexually transmitted diseases, sex yoo all ee trans MIT ud di ZEE zuz
Shaving, SHAY ving
Shingles, SHIN gulz
Shivering, SHIV uh ring
Shock, SHAHK
Shyness, SHYE nus
Sickle-cell anemia, SIK ul-sel uh NEE mee uh
Sight, SYTE
Silicosis, sil uh KOH sis
Sinusitis, sye nuh SYTE is
Skeletal system, SKEL uh tul SIS tum
Smallpox, SMAWL pahks
Sodium, SOH dee um
Solvent abuse, SAHL vunt uh BYOOHS
Spina bifida, SPYE nuh BI fuh duh
Spinal column, SPYE nul KAH lum
Spinal cord, SPYE nul KORD
Spine, SPYNE
Spleen, SPLEEN
Sprains, SPRAYNZ
Squint, SKWINT
Stammering and stuttering, STAM uh ring and STUT uh ring
Starch, STAHRCH
Starvation, stahr VAY shun
Stomach, STUM uk
Strep throat, STREP THROTE
Sty, STYE
Substance abuse, SUB stuns uh BYOOS
Suffocation, suf uh KAY shun
Sugar, SHOOG ur
Suicide, SOOH uh syde
Sulfonamides, sul FAHN uh meydz
Sweat, SWET
Symptoms, SIMP tumz

T

Tapeworm, TAYP wurm
Taste, TAYST
Tattooing, ta TOOH ing
Tay-Sachs disease, TAY-SAKS di ZEEZ
Temperature, TEM pruh choor
Tendon, TEN dun

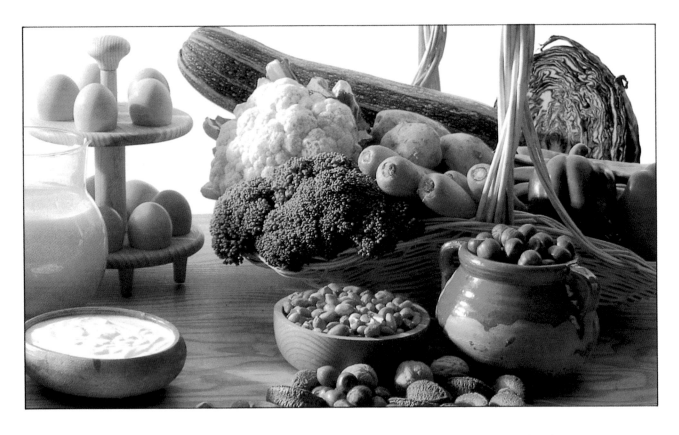

Tension, TEN shun
Tetanus, TET un us
Thalassemia, tha luh SEE mee uh
Thrombosis, thrahm BOH sis
Thymus, THYE mus
Thyroid gland,
  THYE royd GLAND
Tick, TIK
Tissues, TISH ooz
Tongue, TUNG
Tonsils and tonsillitis, TAHN sulz
  and TAHN suh LYE tis
Tourette's syndrome, tooh RETS
  SIN drohm
Tourniquet, TOOR ni kay
Toxic shock syndrome, TOK sik
  SHAHK SIN drohm
Tranquilizers,
  TRANG kwuh lye zerz
Transfusion, trans FYOOH shun
Transplants, TRANS plants
Trench mouth, TRENCH mowth
Trichinosis, trik uh NOH sis
Trypanosomiasis,
  tri PAN uh soh MEYE uh sis
Tuberculosis, too bur kyuh LOH sis
Tularemia, too luh REE mee uh
Tumor, TOOH mur

Tunnel vision, TUH nul VIZH un
Typhoid fever, TYE foyd FEE vur
Typhus, TYE fus

U

Ulcer, UL sur
Unconsciousness,
  un KAHN shus nus
Urethra, yoo REE thruh
Urethritis, yoo ree THRYE tis
Urinary system, YOOR un ner ee SIS
  tum
Urticaria, ur ti CAHR ee uh
Uterus, YOOHT ur us

V

Vaccination, vak suh NAY shun
Vagina, vuh JYE nuh
Varicose veins, VAR uh kohs VAYNZ
Vegetarianism,
  veg uh TAR ee uh ni zum
Vein, VAYN
Venereal diseases, vuh NIR ee ul
  di ZEE zuz
Ventricular fibrillation,
  ven TRIK yuh lur
  fib ruh LAY shun
  (*or* FYE bruh lay shun)

Vertigo, VURT uh goh
Virginity, vur JIN uh tee
Viruses, VYE rus is
Vitamins VYTE un minz
Vomiting, VAH muh ting

W

Wart, WAWRT
Water pollution, WAWT ur
  puh LOO shun
Weight control, WAYTE kun trohl
Weil's disease, VEYLZ di ZEEZ
Whiplash injury, HWIP lash
  IN jur ee
Whooping cough, HOOP ping
  KAWF
Withdrawal symptoms,
  with DRAW ul SIM tumz
Worms, WURMZ
Wounds, WOOHNDZ

XYZ

X ray, EKS-ray
Yoga, YOH guh

Health Organizations, Websites, and Hot Lines

The health organizations listed here are grouped into subject areas for easy reference. Most are nonprofit organizations that provide public information and have chapters throughout the United States. To find a local group, look in the phone book; if none exists in your immediate locality, try the nearest large town or city, or telephone the organization for information. Calls to many hot lines and organizations have numbers beginning 800 and are toll free.

Also included are the e-mail and Website addresses of the oganizations listed here. The Websites provide an overview of the aims of the organization and the various ways in which they can be contacted.

AIDS

Project Inform
205 13th Street, #2001
San Francisco, CA 94103
Tel: (415) 558-8669
Fax: (415) 558-0684
E-mail: web@projectinform.org
Website: www.projinf.org
Current information about AIDS and its treatment are provided.

Addiction

Addiction Search
Website: www.addictionsearch.com
This site provides links to sites about alcoholism, drug treatment, harm reduction programs, referrals, research, and relevant organizations.

Alcoholism

Al-Anon/Alateen
Al-Anon Family Group Headquarters
P.O. Box 862, Midtown Station
New York, NY 10018
Tel: 800-356-9996
E-mail: wso@al-anon.org
Website: www.al-anon.org
Al-Anon groups provide support for families and friends of people aged between 12 and 20 whose drinking affects the lives of those close to them. There are over 75,000 groups covering most cities and towns of the United States and Canada.

Allergies

American Academy of Allergy Asthma & Immunology
611 East Wells Street
Milwaukee, WI 53202
Tel: (414) 272-6071
Patient information and physician referral line: 800-822-2762
E-mail: info@aaaai.org
Website: www.aaaai.org
The AAAAI provides the latest news on asthma and allergies, diet, pollen counts, as well as many other links.

Autism

Autism Society of America
7910 Woodmont Avenue, Suite 300
Bethesda, MD 20814-3067
Tel: (301) 657-0881 or 800-3-AUTISM
Fax: (301) 657-0869
E-mail: info@autism-society.org
Website: www.autism-society.org
The society provides information about autism and the support services that are available to autistic people and their families. It also aims to educate the public about the symptoms of autism and the needs, problems, strengths, and skills of autistic people.

Bereavement

The Compassionate Friends
P.O.Box 3696
Oak Brook, IL 60522
Tel: (630) 990-0010
Fax: (630) 990-0246
E-mail: tcfwebmaster@compassionate friends.org
Website: www.compassionatefriends. org
Parents and children offer support and understanding to other families who have lost a child or sibling. The 600 groups meet monthly and also act as telephone friends.

Birth Defects

March of Dimes Birth Defects Foundation
1275 Mamaroneck Avenue
White Plains, NY 10605
Tel: (888) 663-4637
Fax: (914) 997-4763
Website: www.modimes.org
With offices all over the country, the March of Dimes provides information to the public about birth defects and their prevention. They work with other organizations to establish good care for pregnant women and their babies.

Spina Bifida Association of America
4590 McArthur Blvd. NW, Suite 250
Washington, DC 20007
Tel: 800-621-3141
Fax: (202) 944-3295
E-mail: sbaa@baa.org
Website: www.sbaa.org
This association aims to promote the prevention of spina bifida and to enhance the lives of all affected.

Blindness

American Foundation for the Blind
11 Penn Plaza, Suite 300
New York, NY 10001
Tel: (212) 502-7600
Fax: (212) 502-7777
E-mail: afbinfo@afb. net
Website: www.afb.org
The AFB is an information center for the general public. It records books, conducts public information programs, and operates a large lending library of books for and about blind people.

Cancer

National Cancer Institute
Building 31, Room 10A31
31 Center Drive MSC 2580
Bethesda, MD 20892-2580
Tel: 800-4-CANCER
Website: www.nci.nih.gov
The National Cancer Institute issues information on the different types of cancer and their treatments. It provides support and resources, screening and testing, and publications about cancer and its treatment and prevention. The National Cancer Institute will also supply advice on coping with cancer in daily living.

Deafness

National Association of the Deaf
814 Thayer Avenue
Silver Spring, MD 20910-4500

Tel: (301) 587-1788
Fax: (301) 587-1791
E-mail: NADinfo@nad.org
Website: www.nad.org
The NAD aims to safeguard the accessibility and civil rights of 28 million deaf and hard of hearing Americans in education, employment, health care, and telecommunications. It has expertise in areas such as education, health, employment, rehabilitation, mental health, leadership development, accessibility, and technology.

Diabetes

Juvenile Diabetes Foundation International

432 Park Avenue South
16th Floor
New York, NY 10016-8013
Tel: (212) 785-9500 and 800-223-1138
Website: jdf.usa.com
The Juvenile Diabetes Foundation provides services and support to juvenile diabetics and their families. Educational films and booklets are available to the public.

Disabilities

Learning Disabilities Association

4156 Library Road
Pittsburgh, PA 15234
Tel: (412) 341-1515
Website: www.kidsource.com
The LDA provides services and information to children with learning disabilities and their families. Services include schools, camps, recreation programs, parent education programs, and public interest pamphlets.

National Easter Seal Society

230 West Monroe, Suite 1800
Chicago, IL 60606
Tel: (312) 726-6200
Fax: (312) 726-1494
E-mail: info@easter-seals.org
Website: www.easter-seals.org
850 local chapters of the Easter Seal Society establish and run programs for people with disabilities. They promote integration within the community.

National Information Center for Children and Youth with Handicaps

Box 1492
Washington, DC 20013-1492
Tel: 800-695-0285

Fax: (202) 884-8441
E-mail: nichcy@aed.org
Website: www.nichcy.org
The Center is an information source for families and teachers of children with physical, mental, and emotional disabilities, with the emphasis on education rights and special services.

National Down Syndrome Society

666 Broadway
New York, NY 10012-2317
Tel: 800-221-4602 and (212)-460-9330
Website: www.ndss.org
The society is dedicated to ensuring that people with Down syndrome have the opportunity to achieve their full potential in the community. As well as providing a wide range of information about Down syndrome, the society is involved with education, research, and advocacy on behalf of sufferers.

National Stuttering Association

5100 East La Palma,
Suite 208,
Anaheim Hills,
CA 92807
Tel: 800-364-1677
Fax: (714) 693-7554
E-mail: nsastutter@aol.com
Website: www.nsastutter.org
The 50 groups of the NSA are self-help groups made up of stutterers and their parents and speech pathologists. They also publish brochures and cassettes to educate others about stuttering.

Association For Retarded Citizens

1000 Elmwood Avenue
Rochester, NY 14620
Tel: (716) 271-0660
Website: www.ggw.org/AlSigl/arc
The ARC, both nationally and locally, offers support and information to people with mental retardation and their families. It is also a source of information on mental retardation and its prevention, and also the rights of people with mental retardation.

Diseases

Alzheimer's Association

919 North Michigan Avenue
Suite 1100
Chicago, IL 60611-1676
Tel: (312) 335-8700 and 800-272-3900
Fax: (312) 335-1110

E-mail: info@alz.org
Website: www.alz.org
Families of people with Alzheimer's disease can get information about the condition and support services at this site. They can also get referrals to local organizations that help with daily care.

Arthritis Foundation

P.O. Box 7669
Atlanta, GA 30357-0669
Tel: 800-283-7800
Website: www.arthritis.org
The Arthritis Foundation has a council, the AJAO, that serves the special needs of children, teens, and young adults who have arthritic diseases. They produce a magazine, *Arthritis Today*, which is full of essential information.

United Cerebral Palsy Associations

1600 L Street, NW
Suite 700
Washington, DC 20036
Tel: (202) 776-0406 and 800-872-5827
Fax: (202) 776-0414
E-mail: @ucp.org
Website: www.ucp.org
UCPA has over 200 local chapters that provide services to people with cerebral palsy and their families. They also provide educational literature and other information resources concerning cerebral palsy.

Lupus Foundation of America

1300 Piccard Drive
Suite 200
Rockville, MD 20850-4303
Tel: (301) 670-9292 and 800-558-0121
Website: www.lupus.org
The LFA supplies booklets and fact sheets about lupus to encourage early diagnosis and treatment.

Muscular Dystrophy Association National Headquarters

3300 E. Sunrise Drive
Tucson, AZ 85718
Tel: 800-572-1717
E-mail: mda@mdausa.org
Website: www.mdausa.org
The local chapters of MDA provide services to people with neurological disorders and their families. They support research and provide information about muscular dystrophy and other neurological diseases.

National Multiple Sclerosis Society
733 3rd Avenue
New York, NY 10017
Tel: 800-344-4867
Website: www.nationalmssociety.org
NMSS provides information to
sufferers, their families, and other
interested people. It supports research
to find a cure for MS.

Paget's Disease Foundation
120 Wall Street
Suite 1602
New York, NY 10005-4001
Tel: 800-23-PAGET
Fax: (212) 509-8492
Website: www.paget.org
The PDF supplies information to
professionals, families, and friends of
people with Paget's disease.

**The American Parkinson's Disease
Association**
60 Bay Street, Suite 401
Staten Island, NY 10301
Tel: (718) 988001 and 800-223-2732
Website: www.apdaparkinson.com
The APDA has 47 Information and
Referral Centers, 80 chapters, and
more than 350 support groups
throughout the United States.

**National Reye's Syndrome
Foundation**
426 North Lewis Street,
Bryan, OH 43506,
Telephone: 1-419-636-2679 and 800-
233-7393
Fax: 1-419-636-9897
E-mail: nrsf@reyessyndrome.org
Website: www.reyessyndrome.org
The NRSF provides literature and
information services to help educate
people about Reye's Syndrome.

Drug Addiction
Narcotics Anonymous
PO Box 9999
Van Nuys, CA 91409
Tel: (818) 773-9999 or (818) 773-9999
Fax: (818) 700-0700
E-mail: fsteam@na.org
Website: www.na.org
NA has 5,500 groups throughout the
world. Recovering drug addicts meet
to help each other. Members remain
anonymous and can go to any group.

Eating Disorders
**National Association of Anorexia
Nervosa and Associated Disorders**
PO Box 7
Highland Park, IL 60035
Tel: (847) 831-3438
Fax: (847) 433-4632
E-mail: info@anad.org
Website: www.anad.org
The association provides support, help,
and information to those who are
suffering from eating disorders.

Epilepsy
Epilepsy Foundation of America
4351 Garden City Drive
Landover, MD 20795
Tel: 800-332-1000
E-mail: webmaster@efa.org
Website: www.efa.org
With 85 local chapters, the EFA provides
help and information to people with
epilepsy and their families.

Exceptional Children
Council for Exceptional Children
1920 Association Drive
Reston, VA 22091
Tel: (888) 232-7733
Fax: (703) 264-9494
E-mail: service@cec.sped.org
Website: www.cec.sped.org
The CEC provides information about
children with special education needs.
It also gives advice about the latest
advances in computers, technical
products and programs.

General Health
**American Council on Science and
Health**
1995 Broadway, 2nd Floor
New York, NY 10023
Tel: (212) 362-7044
Fax: (212) 362-4919
E-mail: acsh@acsh.org
Website: www.acsh.org
ACSH provides information on a wide
range of nutritional, environmental,
and related health matters, particularly
AIDS and environmental pollution.

Hemophilia
National Hemophilia Foundation
116 West 32nd Street
11th Floor
New York, NY 10001

Tel: (212) 328-3706
Fax: (212) 328-3788
E-mail: @hemophilia.org
Website: www.hemophilia.org
Hemophiliacs and their families and
professionals make up the volunteer
membership of this organization,
which has 48 local chapters. They
provide services to hemophiliacs and
allow public access to information
about this inherited disease.

Heart and Lung Diseases
American Heart Association
7272 Greenville Avenue
Dallas, TX 75231
Tel: 800-242-8721 or 888-478-7653
Website: www.americanheart.org
The AHA provides information about
the treatment and prevention of heart
disease through free publications and
programs in the community. There are
55 state organizations. At the same
address, Mended Hearts, with 161 local
chapters, is made up of people who
have had heart surgery and their
families and friends, who offer support
to each other. The phone number for
Mended Hearts is (214) 706-1442.

American Lung Association
1740 Broadway
New York, NY 10019
Tel: (212) 315-8700
E-mail: info@lungusa.org
Website: www.lungusa.org/site_index
The ALA is committed to fighting lung
diseases in all its forms, providing a
special emphasis on asthma, tobacco
control, and environmental health.

Home/Hospice Child Care
**Make-A-Wish Foundation
of America**
3550 North Central Avenue
Suite 300
Phoenix, AZ 85012-2127
Tel: (602) 279-9474 or 800-722-9474
Fax: (602) 279-0855
E-mail: mawfa@wish.org
Website: www.wish.org
The purpose of the foundation is to
grant the wish of any life-threateningly
ill child. When doing this, they will pay
for the expenses of the child and family.
The foundation looks at the whole
family when granting wishes.

Children's Hospice International
901 North Pitt Street
Suite 230
Alexandria, VA 22314
Tel: (703) 684-0330 or 800-2-4-CHILD
Fax: (703) 684-0226
E-mail: chiorg@aol.com
Website: www.chionline.org
CHI provides information about support groups and education for people interested in hospice care for children.

Injuries
Phoenix Society for Burn Survivors
2153 Wealthy Street SE, #215
East Grand Rapids, MI 49506
Tel: (616) 458-2773 or 800-888-2876
Fax: (616) 458-2831
E-mail: info@phoenix-society.org
Website: www.phoenix-society.org
With over 60 regional groups, the Phoenix Society is a self-help organization for burn victims and their families. It provides public education about burns and disfigurement and helps children rehabilitate.

The Brain Injury Association
105 North Alfred Street
Alexandria, VA 22314
Tel: (703) 236-6000 or 800-444-6443
Fax: (703) 236-6001
E-mail: FamilyHelpline@biausa.org
Website: biausa.org
The aim of the BIA is to create a better life and future for brain damaged people through research, brain injury prevention, education, and advocacy.

National Spinal Cord Injury Association
6701 Democracy Boulevard
Suite 300-9
Bethesda, MD 20817
Tel: (301) 588-6959
Fax: (301) 588-9414
Website: www.spinalcord.org
The NSCIA has 32 local groups that offer support and information about spinal cord injuries.

Mental Illness
National Alliance for the Mentally Ill
Colonial Place Three
Suite 300
2107 Wilson Blvd.
Arlington, VA 22201

Tel: (703) 524-7600 or 800-950-6264
Fax: (703) 524-9094
Website: www.nami.org
Information about mental illness is available from the 850 local groups of NAMI. Support and services for patients and their families is provided.

Sexual Health
Planned Parenthood Federation of America
810 Seventh Ave.
New York, NY 10019
Tel: (212) 541-7800
Website: www.plannedparenthood.org
The 128 Planned Parenthood affiliates operate 875 health centers in 48 states and the District of Columbia, providing medical services and sex education to nearly five million people each year.

National Lesbian and Gay Health Foundation
1407 S Street NW
Washington, DC 20009
Tel: (202) 939-7880
Fax: (202) 234-1467 (no Website)
The aim of the Foundation is to coordinate educational activities, develop programs, encourage research into gay and lesbian health care issues, and establish a clearing house for gay and lesbian health concerns. It also provides sources of current information about AIDS.

Campaign for Our Children
120 West Fayette Street, Suite 1200
Baltimore, MD 21201
Tel: (410) 576-9015
Website: www.cfoc.org/
CFOC is an organization that encourages sexual abstinence among adolescents and promotes public awareness about preventative health issues that affect young people.

Smoking
Action on Smoking and Health
2013 H Street, NW
Washington, DC 20006
Tel: (202) 659-4310
Website: http://ash.org
ASH works to protect people from the unwanted social and health effects of tobacco smoking. They will send information upon request that gives

details of smoking-related health problems and the legal rights of non-smokers to socialize, work, or eat in a smoke-free environment.

Shelter/Youth Problems
Salvation Army
615 Slaters Lane
P.O. Box 269
Alexandria, VA 22313
Tel: (703) 684-5500
Fax: (703) 684-3478
Website:www.christianity.com/ salvationarmyusa
The Salvation Army is a Christian association that provides services for young people, including food and shelter centers, homes for single mothers, and medical clinics.

Suicide
Suicide Prevention Center
4760 S. Sepulveda Blvd.
Culver City, CA 90230
Tel: (310) 391-1253 (24 hr line)
Website: www.suicidecrisisline.org
The Suicide Prevention Center has over 80 trained volunteers who perform telephone crisis intervention, bereavement support, and community education. The center operates a 24-hour suicide crisis line. The site also provides a link to a depression test to assess someone's risk of committing suicide.

American Association for Suicidology
4201 Connecticut Avenue, NW
Suite 408
Washington, DC 20008
Tel: (202) 237-2280
Hot Line: 800-SUICIDE
Fax: (202) 237-2282
E-mail: ajkulp@suicidology.org
Website: www.suicidology.org
The goal of the American Association for Suicidology is to understand what makes someone want to commit suicide, and to try to prevent suicide. ASS promotes research, public awareness programs, and education and training for professionals and volunteers. There is also a suicide hot line that provides access to trained telephone counselors for 24 hours a day, 7 days a week.

HEALTH ORGANIZATIONS

Health and Human Services

Health care in the United States is supervised by the Department of Health and Human Services. It is the principal agency for providing essential human services, including medical care, community health, food and drug safety, infant and child care and protection, and substance abuse treatment and prevention.

Medicare

Medicare is a federal insurance plan that provides medical care for persons aged 65 and over, and for people disabled for at least two years.

Medicaid

Medicaid is a federal health insurance system for low-income people.

INTERNATIONAL HEALTH ORGANIZATIONS

The World Health Organization

The (WHO) is one of the agencies of the United Nations. It helps countries to improve their own health services, and coordinates world campaigns against disease. WHO was founded in 1948. Its headquarters are in Geneva, with branch offices in the U.S. and five other countries.

World Medical Association

The World Medical Association links the medical associations of different countries. Its aim is to standardize professional conduct for doctors and to exchange ideas. It has regional organizations for Latin America, the Pacific, Africa, Asia, and Europe.

Rockefeller Foundation

The Rockefeller Foundation is a philanthropic organization that sponsors research into disease, especially in developing countries. It was founded by the multi-millionaire industrialist John D. Rockefeller in 1913.

Red Cross

The International Red Cross is an organization dedicated to the care of the sick and wounded, in war and peace. It was founded in 1863 by a young Swiss banker, Jean Henri Dunant, who campaigned to have wounded soldiers treated as neutrals. The American branch was formed in 1881 and has played a major part in many conflicts since then.

OTHER WEBSITES

Chronic illness help
www.smallcomforts.org/

AIDS
www.aids.org

Angioplasty
www.ptca.org

Asthma
www.asthmacontrol.com

Breast ultrasound
www.imaginis.com

Cancer
www.cancerhelponline.org

Diabetes
www.iddtus.org

Eating disorders
www.bodypositive.com

Endometriosis
www.endocenter.org

Facial pain
www.facial-neuralgia.org

General medical information
www.medhelp.org

Genetics
www.geneticalliance.org

Heart disease prevention
www.heartinfo.org

Hepatitis
www.hepfi.org

Mental health
www.mental-health-matters.com

Multiple sclerosis
www.nationalmssociety.org

Sickle-cell disease
www.emory.edu/peds/sickle

Sleep disorders
www.sleepnet.com/disorder

Spinal cord injury
www.spinalcord.uab.edu

Sports medicine
www.sportsmedicine.com

Stroke
www.strokecenter.org

Teen health issues
www.teengrowth.com
www.kidshealth.org

Thyroid disorders
www.thyroidfoundation.org

Women's health
www.4woman.gov

HOT LINES

Al-Anon, Alateen Family Group
Hot Line: 800-344-2666

Eating Disorders
Hot Line: (947)-831-3438

Environmental Health
Hot Line: 800-368-4358

National Cancer Institute
Hot Line: 800-4-CANCER

National Child Abuse
Hot Line: 800-422-4453

National Runaway
Hot Line: 800-231-6946

Sexually Transmitted Diseases
Hot Line: 800-227-8922

Website Sources

Websites frequently change their locations and links. The addresses here are corrrect at time of publication, but if you experience difficulty in locating a site, search again using key words.

Thematic Indexes

Numerals in **boldface** refer to the volume number; numerals following colons refer to page numbers.

PREVENTION AND CURE

HUMAN BEHAVIOR

Comprehensive Index

Numerals in **boldface** refer to the volume number; numerals in *italics* refer to pictures or their captions.

C

E

W

XYZ

Picture Credits

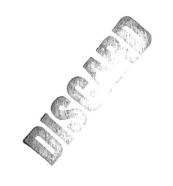